Ecological therapy for Parkinson's disease

(Medication, late and little)

Dr. Rafael González Maldonado
neurologist

Ecological therapy for Parkinson's disease

(Medication, late and little)

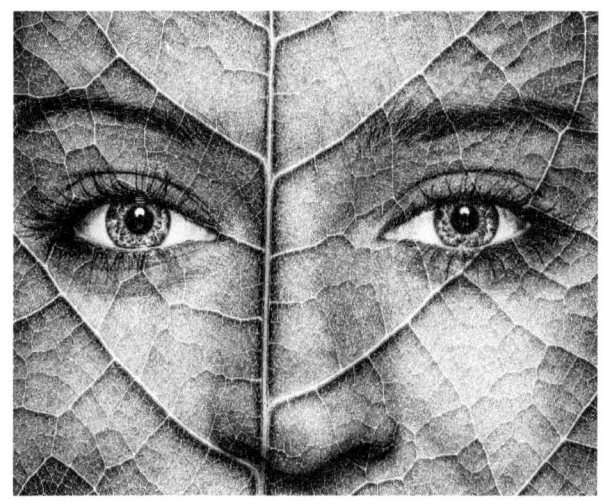

Dr. Rafael González Maldonado
neurologist

Title: Ecological therapy for Parkinson's disease
Subtitle: (Medication, late and little)

Author: Rafael Gonzalez Maldonado

Publisher: KDP Amazon, North Charleston
1st EDITION, February 2023

KDP ISBN: 9798376201596

©*Copyright 2023*: Rafael Gonzalez Maldonado
All rights reserved. rafael@gonzalezmaldonado.com

WARNING: The concepts and data in this book are not medical recommendations but suggestions that are debatabled and subject to error. Patients and their carers should always follow the criteria of their treating physician.

To Yairelis

This simple accident of falling in love is as beneficial as it is astonishing. It arrests the petrifying influence of years, disproves cold-blooded and cynical conclusions, and awakens dormant sensibilities.

(RL STEVENSON, *Virginibus puerisque* 1881)

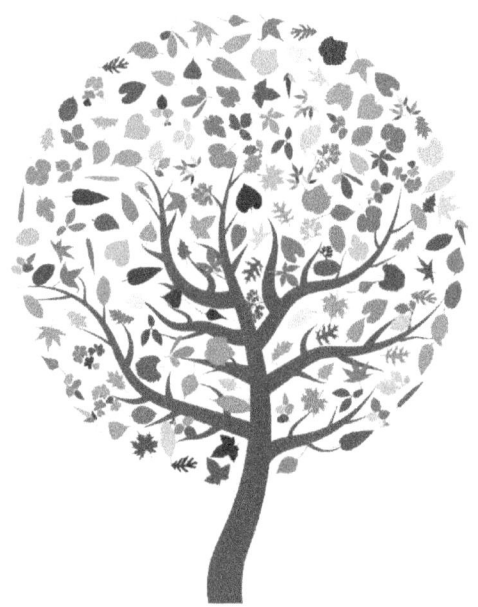

Index

Dedication

Index

Introduction

1. Symptoms Dr. Parkinson never saw
2. Brisk walking instead of Sinemet
3. I feel, therefore I exist
4. Pleasure raises dopamine
5. Stress kills neurons
6. Tell me your dreams and I'll predict your future
7. Parkinson's disease is born in the gut
8. Starting with natural levodopa (mucuna)
9. Mucuna for medicated patients
10. Essential supplements

Bibliography

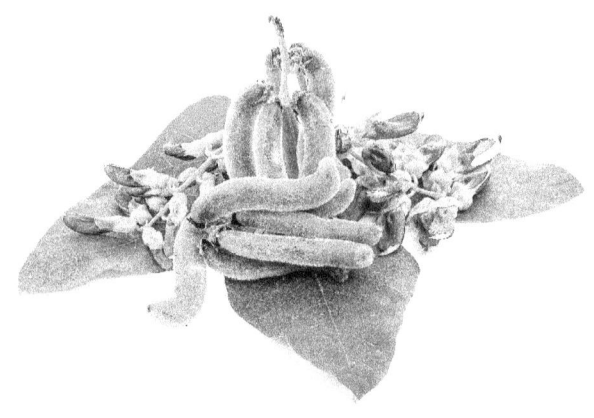

Mucuna pruriens is a tropical bean with a high concentration of levodopa. Its seed powder or extracts are the most effective natural product in the ecological therapy of Parkinson's disease.

Remedies often make troubles worse. Let nature take its course. The wise doctor needs to know when to prescribe something and when not, and often the art lies in not applying any remedy at all

(Baltasar Gracián, 1647)

Introduction

Ecology defends nature from the ravages of man and this *Ecological therapy* aims to protect patients from overmedication.

Five years after diagnosis, they will have two types of symptoms: those of the disease that James Parkinson described and others that the English doctor never saw. These latter are what current drugs cause, at high doses for months and years: dyskinesias, cognitive impairment, syncope, increased constipation, hallucinations, loss of impulse control....

Medications will be necessary at some point, but they should be delayed and given at low doses. In pharmacies you will not find any treatment for Parkinson's disease, only for the symptoms. The evolution does not improve by taking drugs, but quite the opposite: side effects accumulate over time.

Fortunately there are therapies that improve the symptoms and progression of Parkinson's disease, but they are not drugs. Don't look to the pharmacy for what life offers you outside: exercise, pleasure, emotional diet, microbiota, or lifestyle changes will greatly improve you so that you will be able to delay the use of pharmaceuticals. And when levodopa becomes necessary, it is preferable to start with the natural one, the levodopa contained in the seeds of mucuna, a tropical bean that allows you to reduce the doses of Sinemet or Madopar.

This book is not a prescription but information for people interested in Parkinson's disease. It should not be used without the supervision of the regular doctor.

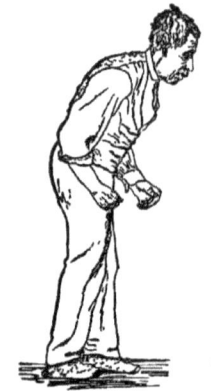

The DISEASE'S OWN symptoms

Tremor

Rigidity

Hipokinesia

Symptoms DUE TO MEDICATION, after 4 years

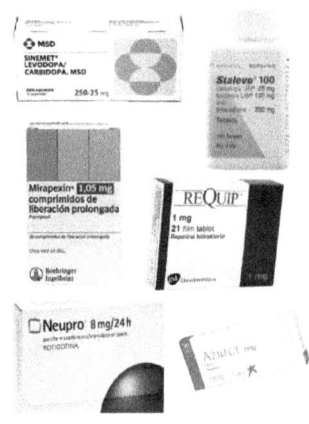

Dyskinesias

Hallucinations

Uncontrolled impulses

Daytime sleepiness

plus Nightmares

plus Constipation

FIGURE 1. After 4-5 years of treatment, the symptoms of Parkinson's disease will be added to those caused by the drugs. Medication should be delayed and given in small doses (*late and little*).

1. Symptoms Dr. Parkinson never saw

James Parkinson never saw dyskinesias... because there was no levodopa. His patients did not hallucinate, nor did they lose control of their impulses, nor did they have nightmares because no one sold pramipexole or ropirinol. Without carbidopa they did not suffer neuropathies, and without rasagiline the heart rhythm was not disturbed.

AT 5 YEARS, NEW SYMPTOMS DUE TO DRUGS

Remedies often make troubles worse.* After five years of treatment, we will see two types of symptoms: those of Parkinson's disease (stiffness, slowness, tremor) and the *new ones* due to many drugs accumulated over months and years.

It is scary to read the prospectuses of antiparkinsonian drugs. They are necessary, they improve symptoms and, sooner or later, they will have to be taken. But they have a less friendly side as the years go by.

In the pharmacy you will not find any treatment for Parkinson's disease, only for the symptoms. If no medication is taken, the disease will follow its natural course. We are not dealing with an infection that requi-

---

* B. Gracián, Spanish philosopher: *Muchas veces empeoran los males con los remedios. Dejar hacer a la naturaleza allí. Tanto ha de saber el sabio médico para recetar como para no recetar, y a veces consiste el arte más en el no aplicar remedios*[89].

res antibiotics against bacterial invasion. With levodopa or pramipexole, mobility and tremor improve, but if you do not take them, the disease will not worsen, rather the opposite.

HE "DANCES" BECAUSE OF TOO MANY PILLS

If a patient moves as if he were dancing, it means that he has too much medication. Levodopa or dopamine agonists, or both, should be reduced.

As these drugs did not exist in James Parkinson's time, his patients did not make these strange, *choreic*, dance-like movements of arms and legs (dyskinesias). Nowadays, patients do not gesticulate by disease but because they were given too many pills. Tremor is something set apart: a *regular* movement, like a pendulum, and its cause would be the opposite: dopamine is lacking, not exceeding.

Dyskinesias and motor fluctuations (oscillations, on-off, end-of-dose phenomenon) appear four to five years after medication. They are more frequent with levodopa but are also seen with dopamine agonists (ropinirole, pramipexole) which add significant side effects: hallucinations, sleep disturbances, severe constipation, daytime sleepiness.

IN PRAISE FOR LEVODOPA

Thanks to levodopa, Parkinson's patients are living better and longer. After fifty years, no drug has been discovered that surpasses its efficacy and tolerance.[262] At some point it has to be given, but the problem is that it causes dyskinesias in the long term and at high doses.

When levodopa reaches the brain, the neurons generate the dopamine that is missing in Parkinson's disease. Dopamine also affects the heart and gut, and early in treatment may cause tachycardia and nausea.

These discomforts decreased when the manufacturers added carbidopa (Sinemet) or benserazide (Madopar) which inhibit the dopa-decarboxylase enzyme*. Sinemet 25/250 has a 1:10 levodopa/carbidopa ratio which was later augmented to 1:4 in Sinemet Plus 25/100 to reduce side effects.

TOO MUCH CARBIDOPA ANTICIPATES DYSKINESIA

The generally accepted assumption is to blame levodopa for dyskinesias and other motor complications. But now some experts now point to decarboxylase inhibitors as the culprits or accomplices: those taking higher ratios of carbidopa (Sinemet Plus) or benserazide (Madopar) will suffer dyskinesias two years earlier.†

Initiating treatment with levodopa there are more side effects and should be combined with more decarboxylase inhibitor (Sinemet Plus 25/100, Madopar 50/200); but soon the patient gets used to it, tolerates it better and

---

* Dopadecarboxylase metabolizes levodopa to dopamine, which irritates the heart and intestines. Carbidopa inhibits dopadecarboxylase, thereby stopping dopamine in the blood but not in the brain, because it does not pass the blood-brain barrier, and it is converted to dopamine there.

† Dyskinesias appear 4 years after taking Madopar or Sinemet Plus (1:4 ratio) and 6 years after taking Sinemet 25/250 (1:10)[9].

needs less carbidopa (Sinemet 25/250). In advanced cases, dyskinesias improve if carbidopa is reduced and even giving only levodopa.[106]

In mucuna there is no carbidopa or benserazide, and perhaps for this reason it hardly generates dyskinesias.

FEW DYSKINESIAS WITH LOW-DOSE LEVODOPA

Dyskinesias due to levodopa are dose dependent. There is less risk of long-term complications if 300-400 mg per day is not exceeded in the first years.[120,128]

At these low doses, leading neurologists prefer levodopa from the start[120,128,150] as an alternative to dopamine agonists, which are less effective and cause interactions and significant side effects.*

For newly diagnosed patients under orthodox treatment, the following is recommended: small doses of synthetic levodopa (less than 300-400 mg per day), combined with a high ratio of carbidopa at the start, which would be lowered when the nausea disappears. And a mixed, more ecological therapeutic option: some of the levodopa should be of natural origin (mucuna).

AGONISTS ARE ANNOYING "ACOLYTES"

Dopamine agonists (ropinirole, pramipexole) mimic the action of levodopa, they are far less efficient, merely *acolytes* or adjuvants that are also annoying. They are

---

* In patients taking levodopa 300 mg daily for 80 weeks, there was no change during the disease[234].

sold with the excuse that levodopa causes dyskinesias* but they also cause them, along with other complications[130,262]: nightmares, REM sleep disorders, visual hallucinations, episodes of confusion, hypersexuality, pathological gambling, compulsive shopping, and other impulse control disorders.

IS IT WORTH TWO YEARS ON AGONISTS?

Ropinirole and pramipexole produce fewer dyskinesias than levodopa but are less effective; most patients do not tolerate them for long† because of the small benefit in relation to the harm they cause. At two or three years they will need to add levodopa.

After five years, those who were maintained with agonists alone have fewer dyskinesias than those treated with levodopa, but a few years later there is no difference, despite having *saved* levodopa.[193] The supposed preventive effect of motor complications does not work.‡ Early treatment with dopamine agonists does not improve the outcome of patients.[206]

---

* The laboratories that sell agonists are the ones that most insisted that levodopa produces dyskinesias.

† An increasing number of patients are refusing treatment with agonists., half of them give up before one year.[68,192]

‡ Taking only agonists results in fewer dyskinesias, but soon levodopa must be added. Over time they will be the same as if they had taken levodopa... and they will have lost years of quality of life.

CONSTIPATED, NIGHTMARES AND DAYTIME SLEEPINESS

Years before the motor symptoms, patients are constipated, but it is aggravated by medication, especially dopamine agonists.[165]

Half of Parkinson's patients are daytime sleepy.[209] This is favoured by the disease in which sleep nerve centres (locus ceruleus) degenerate, but with treatment, daytime sleepiness* increases, especially with agonists and benzodiazepines. And when sleep is disturbed, cognitive and motor development worsens.

All dopamine agonists impair sleep and decrease REM (when most dreaming occurs), almost from the are start.[27] Ropinirole is the one with the greatest nocturnal sleep impairment, the highest daytime sleepiness, and the earliest dyskinesias.[131]

TRAFFIC ACCIDENTS DUE TO AGONISTS

If you had a traffic accident because you suddenly fell asleep while driving, it is the fault of pramipexole or ropinirole; it has happened before.[31] I am not talking about the usual daytime drowsiness but about dangerous and sudden sleep attacks that are unpredictable.[22,31,255]

All agonists (ropinirole, pramipexole, and also the ergotics no longer in use) can trigger sleep attacks,[22,171,255] sometimes without warning of previous diurnal somno-

---

* In the description of James Parkinson (*An essay on the shaking palsy* 1817)[168] only one case with sleep problems is mentioned, which he attributes to the fact that rigidity and tremors do not allow him to sleep.

lence. The risk increases with high doses and long treatments; it is lower with levodopa and others.[171,255]

WATCH YOUR HEART AND BLOOD PRESSURE: MAOI*

MAOI (selegiline, rasagiline and safinamide) favour hypotensive or hypertensive crises and distort heart rhythm. They alleviate daytime sleepiness but worsen sleep at night. Some people *need* rasagiline because they move less when it is withdrawn, but this does not compensate for the benefit/detriment ratio, except in some young people and specific cases.

When a patient becomes dizzy when standing up, it is usually due to orthostatic hypotension, sometimes leading to syncope. This is caused by the disease but is aggravated by MAOIs, levodopa, agonists, and general medication†.

Some publications show a slight increase in mortality in patients taking MAO-B inhibitors compared with those treated with agonists. And this is worse when they were given com-bined with other drugs. There is a higher risk in men, in older people and in those with high blood pressure or heart problems.[231]

---

* MAOI are drugs that inhibit monoamine oxidase: selegiline (Plurimen), rasagiline (Azilect) and safinamide (Xadago).

† Blood pressure decreases as Parkinson's disease progresses, and more so with their medications, with a risk of syncope. Some who were previously hypertensive should reduce hypotensive drugs.

DOPAMINE DEMONS INVADE THE SHY PATIENT

All his life he was so shy and quiet and now he thinks himself the best in the world, is obsessed with shopping and sex, he tries to flirt with anyone, invents fantastic businesses and he could bet all his money in the casino. He is a different person... since that treatment.

We are dealing with a lack of impulse control, what Dr. Lees called *the dopamine demons*.[59] Too much medication burden leads to dopaminergic dysregulation syndrome.

The usual culprits are dopamine agonists, sometimes early and at low doses: one patient who started on minimal intake of pramipexole (0.18 mg) quickly developed pathological gambling and hypersexuality.[51]

A variant that may go unnoticed is the so called *punding*: I have not found an appropriate translation into Spanish or French: it consists of stereotyped behaviour, with automatic motor rituals, in which the patient engages in repeatedly assembling and dissembling objects, gathering them up or classifying them.[8]

IF HALLUCINATIONS, REMOVE ALL EXCEPT LEVODOPA

Antiparkinsonian drugs can produce visual hallucinations, especially pramipexol and other dopamine agonists.[123,180] Also, there are cases of delirium, psychosis and mania due to amantadine.[154]

Psychiatric pathology follows a defined sequence: they start with sleeping problems (insomnia, nightmares, agitation); then come vivid dreams, hallucinations, delusions and culminate in psychosis.[123] As soon as this chronology is detected, all antiparkinsonian drugs except levodopa should be reduced or withdrawn.

WHY DO PATIENTS NOW DIE EARLIER?

Levodopa was a revolutionary treatment (since the 1960s) that allowed patients to live longer and better. Half a century later, the new drugs have not revolutionised anything.

By coincidence or not, mortality from Parkinson's disease, which had been falling dramatically, is rising in recent years, precisely when patients have more doctors and new drugs are available.

Since 1999, more patients of all races and ages, but more white men, have been dying in the United States.[198] The same is reported in Spain, England, Australia[182] and other countries.* It could be attributed to higher incidence or to the fact that Parkinson's disease is now more widely coded as a cause of death,[38] but there are other views†.

The data are clear although interpretations vary. Some suggest that polypharmacy improves their quality of life but shortens it: patients would live better... for fewer years.

---

* In Spain, deaths from Parkinson's disease increased dramatically (by 78 %) from 2006 (2,508 deaths) to 2018 (4,483).[264] In England, they also increased between 2001 and 2014.

† DBS (deep brain stimulation) patients live longer, so some assume that it is neuroprotective. Others suggest that the *protection* has a simple explanation: as they need fewer drugs, they are less damaged by them.

LABORATORIES PAY FOR CLINICAL TRIALS

I do not question the honesty of the pharmaceutical industry, but the most widespread clinical trials are those designed, ordered, sponsored, and published by the laboratories, on the medicines they sell. And of course, the most favourable results are those that are submitted to journals and congresses. Negative findings are less often reported.[128]

Trials are usually conducted with average patients. Complicated or advanced cases are not included, nor are those over 75 years of age, nor those with heart problems or polypathologies.[149] The adverse effects of medication in such people are not sufficiently studied, and they will then be prescribed those drugs that may actually be detrimental to them.[128]

IF A DRUG DID NOT IMPROVE YOU, QUIT IT

No pharmaceuticals cure Parkinson's disease, they are merely optional, only for the symptoms. Therefore, if a drug bothers you, ask your doctor how you can withdraw it. The same if it doesn't annoy you, but you don't get better.

Another fundamental rule to be *negotiated* with your doctor: delay medication as long as you can and, when you need it, take as little as possible: *medication, late and little*.

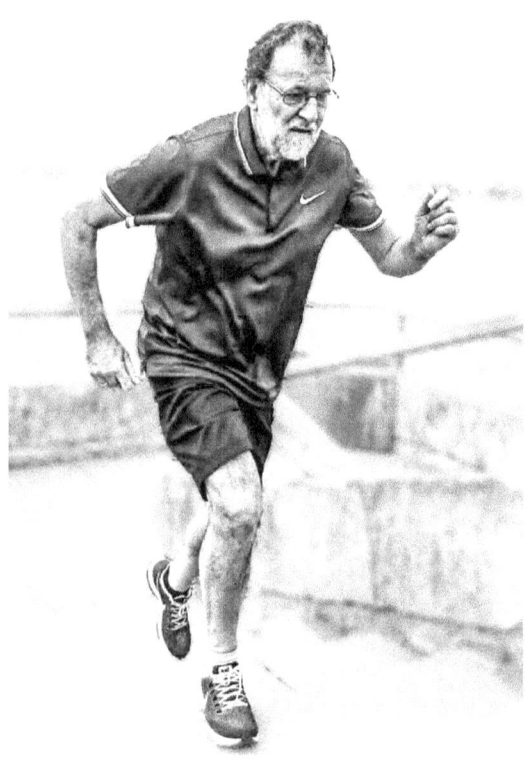

FIGURE 2: Brisk walking (quick steps, exaggerated arm movements) is the exercise that increases dopamine levels the most. We used to see it on television when Mariano Rajoy, then president of Spain, appeared on television practising sport.

2. Brisk walking instead of Sinemet

Walking fast and outdoors is the best treatment for Parkinson's disease. No drug will prevent it from progressing. There is only one remedy to slow its course: exercise, physical activity.[57]

THE SOFA PREDISPOSES TO PARKINSON'S DISEASE

Long hours on the couch contribute to Parkinson's disease: at the time of diagnosis, most patients are sedentary.[135] People who move around get less Parkinson's [60,210,226] and less Alzheimer's.[97] You may protect yourself from these pathologies by walking, swimming, or doing sport: get moving! Life is movement.

There are two types of evolution in patients: 1) those who do not walk will get worse and die earlier, and 2) those who move frecuently will delay the disease and live longer and better.[251]

EXERCISE SLOWS PARKINSON'S DISEASE

Exercise reduces motor symptoms, clears the mind, and slow down Parkinson's pathology because it stimulates the plasticity of neurons in the corticostriatal and cognitive circuits.[114] Being in motion raises brain dopamine and protects neurons, as seen in mice and tested in patients.* A single session of aerobic exercise enhances neuroplasticity and motor learning.[28]

BRISK WALKING (RAJOY'S MARCH)

What raises dopamine the most is brisk walking, whether or not you have Parkinson's. Walking is good, running is good, but it is better if you walk accelerating the pace and moving the arms exaggeratedly.[138] As in good cars, more important than speed is *reprise*, the ability to accelerate in a few seconds.

Do you remember Mariano Rajoy when, as president of Spain, he appeared walking quickly and waving his arms around? The *march of Rajoy* is the best treatment. You should walk briskly several times a day and within a week you will notice the benefit. Ten minutes of brisk walking is better than an hour's walk… or half a Sinemet tablet.

RAPID AND BRIEF VIGOROUS EXERCISE

Instead of many steps, rather than a long promenade, go for a brisk walk. And better if you add a few minutes of *short vigorous exercise*, such as sprinting after a runaway bus, or quickly climbing stairway. It is this brief, fast, high-intensity activity that most improves Parkinson's patients.[103,133]

Three minutes of strenous exercise is equivalent to the famous 10,000 steps a day.[217]

---

* *Parkinsonised* mice retain dopamine if they run on a treadmill.[227,228] For patients, everyone recommends physical activity,[195,205,207,225] which protects dopaminergic neurons[161] and induces growth factors.[203,263]

Indoors you could also walk up the stairs rapidly (if there is no risk of falling), several times a day, carrying a backpack with a small load (or without it). This raises dopamine (and testosterone in men), increases your daily well-being, and will extend your lifespan.[71] Please step down carefully.

WALKING WITH MUSIC AND SMART GLASSES

In Parkinson's disease, the kinetic melody, the *music* of movement, the panache, is lost. To help your gait, you can steal the rhythm you lack from music: try dancing or walking wearing headphones, while a military march, Wagner's *Ride of the Valkyries* or any upbeat song is playing. You will move faster, sleep better, be lively and more active in everyday tasks.[53,118,153,197,245]

Acoustic (with music or a metronome), visual (lines on the floor) and tactile (a bar on the corridor wall) cues can be installed at home to prevent gait blocks, adapting to each patient.[250]

Advanced technology is being developed with Android smart glasses that provide the patient with multi-sensory cues: acoustic (music and rhythms), visual (images) and haptic (tactile), which are coordinated to facilitate walking and avoid blockages.[111]

IF WALKING IS PAINFUL, IT'S TIME TO SWIM

Some patients cannot walk as much as they would like because of knee or hip pain. This is the time for swimming. In therapeutic natation there is no pain in the legs because they are not bearing weight.

Patients will be controlled by a monitor and, no matter how well they can swim, they are fitted with a life jacket. This way they do not waste time and strength trying to float; they are sure not to sink and they will move freely in the water, like in a ballet.

The result is spectacular. Swimming develops mobility, gait, and balance (thus reducing falls) as much or more than land-based exercises.[23,112]

DYSKINESIAS ARE REDUCED BY SWIMMING

Swimming requires harmonising the movements of the limbs in a complex synergy and is used as a natural treatment for ataxias and other coordination problems.[248] It has also been found to improve dyskinesias; this was an unexpected finding in people with intensive aquatic activities over several weeks.[195]

THE "MOTOR MEMORY" OF GAIT

The novice falls off the bike because he has not automated pedalling with body weight and balance. Learning creates new neural circuits that are stored as *motor memory*.

In Parkinson's patiens the motor memory of gait declines. They *forgot* to walk with coordinated movements of the limbs and it is difficult for them to take long strides; nervous circuits were blurred in the gait, which becomes slow, without automatisms, like a robot, graceless.

There are physiotherapists specialised in recovering this automatic gait, and many Parkinson's associations have them. The patient is trained to learn to walk again. As in football: to know how to take a penalty kick, you must repeat it, until the neurons automate the appropriate circuits, and imprint the new skill in motor memory.

ANY EXERCISE IMPROVES PATIENTS

Nordic walking, aided by the impulse of poles (similar to those used in skiing), is an outdoor endurance sport, very effective and beneficial.[99]

Exercising on a stationary bike is very positive, and even more so on a touring cycle, provided there is no risk of falling.[199] Innovatively, some physiotherapists train with virtual reality before exercises, with good results in gait and balance.[62]

Mind control techniques are very helpful for people with Parkinson's disease.[113,125,237]. Tai-chi encourages gait, adds quality of life, relieves fatigue and depression, clarifies the mind and favours sleep.[237]

A GARDEN, A PARK, A FOREST

We need plants and trees around us. If you open your window and see only buildings, go to the park, every day.

Gait blocking increases in enclosed or urban spaces and decreases in the open air, walking in contact with nature.[160] Don't get on a treadmill in the gym, with air conditioning and wireless headphones. Run in the countryside, in the fresh air, feeling the sun, hearing the birds. Spending time outdoors is a wise and great treatment for Parkinson disease.[236]

CITIZENS HAVE DIVORCED FROM NATURE

The civilised world is divorced from nature, in artificial environments. The romantic Wordsworth long ago complained*: *Getting and spending we lay waste our powers; little we see in Nature that is ours.*

Parkinson's is a disease of the civilised world, an advancing pandemic. In the 19th century this pathology was a rarity and, by 2040, 17 million patients are expected. It is a result of the *advances* of civilisation: pesticides, industrial products, processed foods, electronic screens everywhere, sedentary lifestyles and general lifestyle.

Digital technology has transformed the way we live and communicate, and that is changing our brains.[213] There are psychological and social costs for young people and adults: attention deficit, cognitive disorders (digital fog, *techno-brain* burnout, overload (inefficient multitasking), addictions (*screen-sucking,* online-compulsive disorder) and, of course, *techno-stress.*[213]

THE WISE HAVE A GARDEN

For millennia, wise people have felt the need for contact with nature, for the energy it gives them.

Shamans seek remote places, yogis go to the forest, Christian fathers retreat to the deserts, and American Indians seek natural visions. They experience nature as

---

*Wordsworth, *The world is too much with us*, 1807.[244]

healing and calming, removing mental trivia, and reminding us of what really matters.

Philosophers and writers verified it: *If next to the library you have a garden, you already have everything** said Cicero. And Fray Luis de León† boasted:

An orchard I have made with my own hand / that in the sweet springtide / all in fair flower doth stand.

Nature is a powerful therapy for Parkinson's disease which promotes well-being, and effectively regenerates motor and cognitive functions, at no cost and without side effects.[12]

TRUE TREATMENT IS A LIFESTYLE CHANGE[236]

We get sick as we live. The good news is that we also heal if we change the way we live : with exercise, nutrition and diet, entertainment, relationships, relaxation and stress management, religious or spiritual involvement, and service to others.[236]

Life is change. Try different exercises, meet new friends, discover fun hobbies, follow alternative routes, go to unfamiliar places.

This is neuroplasticity: as events in your life change, neurons in your brain form new connections, which improve your movements and your memory. There are

---

* *Si hortum in bibliotheca habes, deerit nihil* (Cicero, 106-43 BC).[33]

† In his "Vida retirada" ("To retired life"), Fray Luis de León discovers the contact with nature: ... *del monte en la ladera, por mi mano plantado tengo un huerto, que con la primavera de bella flor cubierto....*

classic studies comparing the neuroimaging and mental capacity of bus drivers (same vehicle, same route) with that of taxi drivers (variable routes) in London: the latter, who travel thousands of streets, excel in cognitive tests and develop more neurons in their hippocampus.[91,137]

Lifestyle change is a very successful treatment for Parkinson disease. Be brave!

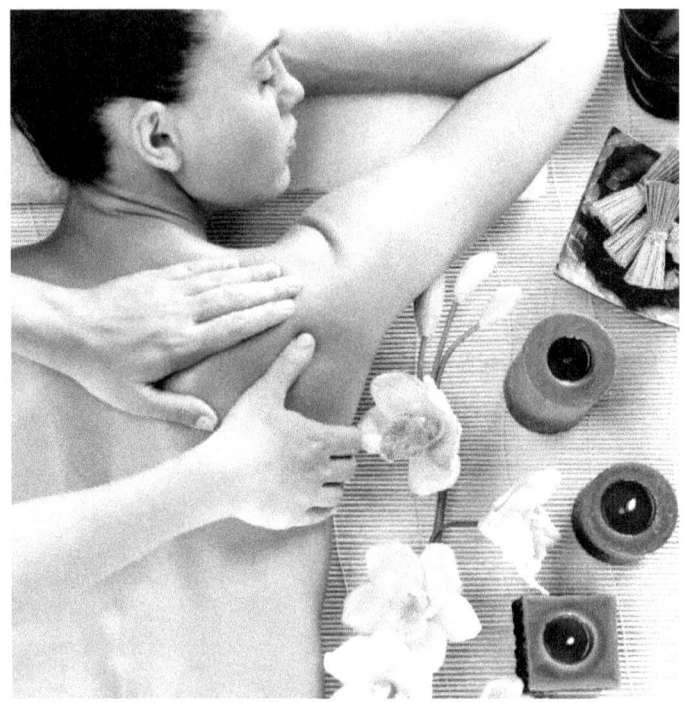

FIGURE 3: Sensory diet nourishes the brain: colours, smells, tastes, caresses, music. Massage is a sensory luxury that empower patients.

3. I feel, therefore I exist*

Sensory nerves are the roots that nourish the brain. It is enough to touch a parkinsonian patient to relieve or even break his blockage. The body must be touched, caressed, massaged; a flood of sensations will be extremely valuable for people with Parkinson disease.[86]

SENSORY DIET

The diet of the senses is more important than the diet of food.[84] Stomachs are fed with potatoes and meat, but the nervous system is nourished by sensory stimuli: the brain thrives on colours, smells, tastes, caresses and sounds. Without them, it atrophies, shrivels, shrinks.

Parkinsonian patients are rarely caressed, and they avoid *rubbing* (physically and mentally) with others. Many keep their minds controlled and controlling, ruled by reason, but they have forgotten their bodies, as if they were unaware that they have flesh and bones, that those muscles and limbs belong to them, and that they deserve attention and care.

The body exists, it is ours, and we must enjoy it, touch it, fondle it. Touch contributes to the *sensory diet* with massages, caressing, and fondling. Nervous nutrition is enhanced when massages are accompanied by music,

---

* With his famous *Cogito ergo sum* ("I think therefore I exist") Descartes praised Reason. "I feel, therefore I exist" (*Sentio ergo sum*) highlights the advantages of feeling and emotion... particularly for parkinsonian patients.

aromas, flavours, and colours. A good massage restores our communication with the body and the senses.

FEELING IS LIFEBLOOD FOR THE BRAIN

The brain grows at the expense of sensation. The occipital lobe (the seat of vision) atrophies if light does not reach it. If you leave a newborn rat in the dark, that part of its brain degenerates, shrinks. You could give it all the vitamins or nutrients, or whatever, but its neurons weaken and die.

Light and colours nourish the occipital lobe, smells and tastes make the hindbrain grow, caresses nurture the parietal cortex, and music and poetry develop the temporal region. All these sensations and senses also leave their mark on the limbic (emotional) system and the base ganglia (the movement nuclei). Feeling is the brain's lifeblood.

CHARCOT'S VIBRATORY CHAIR

Charcot was a neurologist, French and very observant. He noticed that his patients improved after a long train journey, sitting in those shaking 19th century carriages, lacking shock absorbers. He attributed it to the rattling whose vibratory sensations, which ascended through the passengers' spinal cords to feed the brain nuclei damaged by the disease.

He then invented his famous *chaise trépidant*: a chair that vibrated with gears and levers that he connected to it. With the patient seated, an assistant turned the handle, and the mechanism made it move with a peculiar jiggle, imitating that of those trains.

A TRACTOR RIDE BEFORE THE SINEMET

This story was told to me by a colleague (and good friend) and I published[80] it in 1997: now I realise that it was the past century, how time flies! His parkinsonian patient claimed to get better in the mornings because, before Sinemet, he used to take a tractor ride.

It seemed silly to us until we related it to old trains and Charcot's chair. The rattling of the tractor mobilises the joints, mechanically relaxes the muscles, and stimulates the vibratory, proprioceptive sensitivity, which reaches the brain via the posterior tracts of the spinal cord. These vibratory stimuli are a *sensory diet* for the neurons and movement *nuclei*.

STABILITY-ENHANCING VIBRATIONS

The hustle of Charcot's *rattling* chair or the tractor ride had a basis in fact: now rehabilitators use body-transmitted vibrations to regenerate stability in parkinsonian patiens.[54,200]

Whole body vibration is a generic term for mechanical oscillations that are transferred to the human organism. They are seen in everyday life (when sitting on a train or tractor) and in some jobs (use of pneumatic hammers). Under expert supervision, body vibration applied during regular physical exercise is beneficial, increases bone density and improves postural stability.[54,117,200]

In other modern variants, they are trained on vibrating platforms, or vibrations and pressure are applied to the soles of the feet and this sensory feedback enhances the walking movement and blockages decrease by 60%.[177]

SENSORY DISCHARGES IMPROVE MOTOR CONTROL

Voluntary movements require coordination with the sensory system. Sensory discharges in the skin, muscles and joints reach the brain and activate motor neurons to enhance movement control; this is how dyskinesias are treated after a stroke[32], and also similarly in Parkinson's patients: sensory-motor entrainment improves motor coordination in the upper limbs.[224] Electroacupuncture* is another useful variant of sensory stimulation.[247]

KEEP YOUR FEET ON THE GROUND: "EARTHING".

Primitive man walked barefoot, his feet felt the grass of the field or the sand on the seashore. Then sandals and shoes were invented, and the soles and toes lost their contact with Mother Earth, the goddess Gaea. *Earthing* (connecting with the earth) is what the English call this tendency to walk with bare feet, a return to man's original state, and they claim to feel regenerated.

It is a primitive, telluric sensation that the brain is surely delighted by. Try a barefoot walk on the beach or in the countryside.

---

* Electroacupuncture applies micro-electrical shocks to traditional acupuncture needles and is beneficial for Parkinson's patients.[247]

THUMB SUCKING AND TONGUE KISSING

The sensations that reach the cortex of the brain occupy larger or smaller areas depending on where they come from. The mouth and the hand have many more neurons in the parietal lobe because they are more sensitive. That is why a cut on the lips or thumb hurts more than a cut on the back or toes. For the very same reason, caresses on the mouth and hands are especially pleasant and rewarding.

A baby's brain is stimulated by sucking the thumb, and the neurons of people in love are excited when they kiss, and even more so if they do it with tongue. Kiss a lot, that's sensory diet and brain nourishment.

MASSAGE FOR PARKINSONIAN PATIENTS

Get a massage, at least once a week, and you will realize how great you feel. Massage is a very fruitful sensory diet, highly recommended in Parkinson's disease[140]: combined with essential oils and music, prevents stiffness, and maintains mobility.

Kneading the muscles reduces contractures and bradykinesia, relieves the fatigue that follows tremors[21], reduces stress, facilitates sleep and gives a general feeling of well-being.[49,223] Persuade your partner to learn how to massage you, and add caresses, even if his or her technique is not professional, you will be charmed.

AROMATHERAPY IN PARKINSON'S

Odours are part of the *sensory diet*. Babies recognise their mothers because they smell them, some aromas trigger old memories, there are perfumes that make people fall in love, and migraine suffereds avoid strong odors. Smell is the shortest and quickest route to the brain.[55,98,191] The olfactory nerve is not a nerve but an extension of the brain that goes directly to the rhinencephalon and the limbic system (where emotion and memory are housed).*

Aromatherapy is a treatment with aromas and fragances, used alone or applied during the massage. Parkinson's patients experience emotional well-being, their body balance is restored, and other symptoms are alleviated.[64]

THE BONBON IS A SENSORY LUXURY

Because of their taste and texture, chocolate bonbons convey a feeling of luxury and pleasure that invades us emotionally: they are a feast for the senses, somewhat hedonic, that provides wellbeing and releases endorphins (our internal morphines).

A good wine with pleasant companionship is another *sensory diet* that the sybarite appreciates. In *gourmet* or *delicatessen shops* you will find luxuries for the taste that raise dopamine and keep away anhedonia (a low capacity for enjoyment), even if you then have to compensate for the calories with exercise. Don't overindulge in these tasty treats.

---

* Proust (*In search of lost time*) narrates that, when as an adult, he smells and savors his famous madeleine, he intensely reminds childhood scenes that he thought forgotten: a certain aroma brings back memories that were stored in his presence.[183]

MOZART REDUCES CORTISOL AND STRESS

"The world without music would be an error" (Nietzsche) and in the Bible music appears as a treatment: David plays the harp to cure Saul *(Samuel 1, 16:23)*. Music modifies moods, controls behaviour, promotes motor skills and helps the well-being of human beings.

Music appears as a treatment in the Bible, when David played the harp to cure Saul (Samuel 1, 16:23). Music modifies moods, controls behaviour, promotes motor skills and helps people's well-being. It can relax us or make us more alert; we can distinguish this by measuring cardiovascular and respiratory responses).

Listening to music* reduces plasma cortisol and lowers blood pressure and heart rate. Fast rhythms keep our attention focused, while slower tempos or pauses relax us.[14]

In Parkinson's patients, music restructures damaged brain functions and encourages emotional and motor responses by combining rhythms, movements and various sensory pathways. The rhythm of music synchronises muscle movements, decreases hypokinesia and bradykinesia, increases motor skills and quality of life.[163,164]

---

* Mozart (Symphony 40) relaxes more than Strauss (*Wiener Blut* : Viennese Blood) and much more than the Abba pop (*Thank you for the Music*).

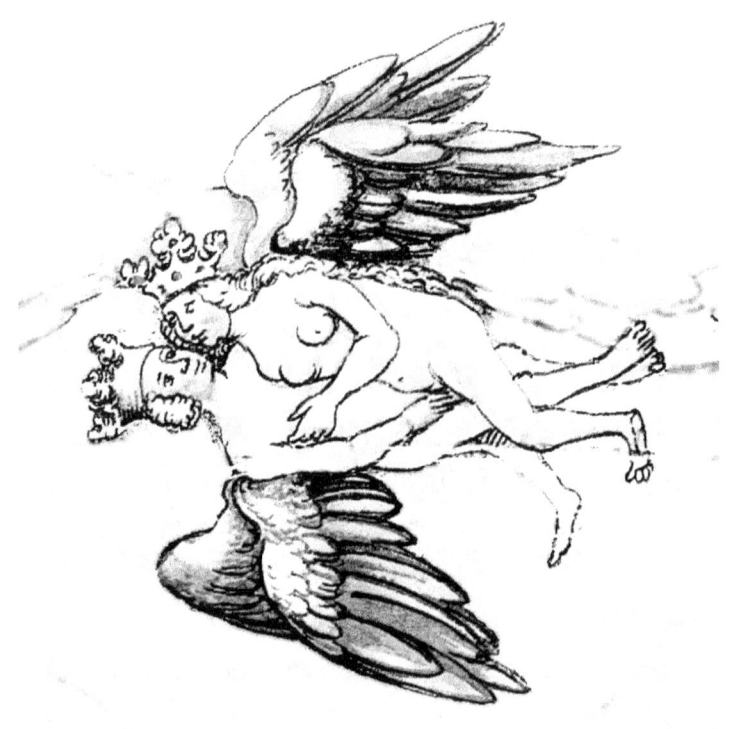

FIGURE 4. Pleasure seeking generates a natural dopamine in the brain that the patient should exploit before increasing the dose of Sinemet.

4. Pleasure raises dopamine

Dopamine is lacking in Parkinson's patients. This neurotransmitter is related to pleasure and, more precisely, it drives the desire or pursuit of pleasure, the motivation to achieve rewards such as sex or food.

If you win the lottery, if your football team is victorious, if you fall in love or if you are awarded a medal, dopamine surges and the symptoms of Parkinson's improve.

PLEASURE IS A PRIMORDIAL FORCE

"All our actions are aimed at increasing pleasure', said Epicurus, and Freud agreed (of course). Pleasure in Greek mythology is represented by Eros* as the primordial source of life.

The pursuit of pleasure generates a natural dopamine in the brain that the patient should take advantage of before increasing the dose of Sinemet. Desire, appetites (at the table or on the bed), the motivation for a voyage, the seeking of novelty or adventure, are all sources of dopamine.

This inclination to enjoyment is what characterises the hedonic personality (*hedon*=pleasure), which causes dopamine to surge, contrary to the attitude of the parkin-

---

* Eros is a pre-Olympian god, a primordial force, the origin of life; he is to be distinguished from his Roman equivalent Cupid, a syrupy and childish image of love.

sonian patient, usually anhedonic, not very plea-sure inclined.

HEDONISM MEANS ENJOYMENT

Hedonism (the capacity and aptitude for enjoyment) depends on dopamine nerve circuits involved in psychological reward mechanisms. Precisely these areas degenerate in Parkinson's disease. In these patients, hedonic tone is diminished[179], and enjoyment and pleasure-seeking behaviour must be encouraged[147].

Just distract yourself with a video game and the striatum releases more dopamine.[122] There are many types of pleasure: intellectual (crossword puzzles), artistic (painting, poetry), social (professional recognition), but the one that boost dopamine the most are the primary ones: food, sex. Rewards, congratulations, medals that we receive, also produce dopamine.

THEY ENJOY LITTLE AND CONTROL A LOT

There is a typical personality before diagnosis. Usually, this patient is orderly, rigidly moral, serious, not impulsive, frugal, quiet, introverted, not very aggressive, cautious, conventional, uptight and perfectionist.

Although shy, he inserts himself socially well, too well, he is a social hyper-adapted person: he easily accepts ethical or group norms, defends them and is inflexible in demanding their fulfilment. The Parkinsonian seeks rules, patterns of behaviour, he craves for the Tables of the Law.[80]

It is assumed that this personality is a consequence of the disease, but it seems that it also influences its evolution, that this lifestyle atrophies the dopaminergic circuits of motivation-pleasure-reward, and that maintaining a psycho-rigid and anhedonic attitude worsens the symptoms and the disease itself. Sad and pessimistic people evolve worse than the optimistic, carefree, and joyful ones.

DR. FAUSTO GIVE UP STUDIES

Dr. Faust (Goethe's) has had enough of books, has wasted too much time studying, and wants to enjoy life again: *All theory is gray, my friend. But forever green is the tree of life**. Immersed in so many books, he forgot to live, and now he regrets it.

That is a good recipe for patients, to exchange knowledge for life: do less *curriculum*, and more biography: dare to live†. It is difficult to change the personality at a certain stage of life, but psychotherapy should promote a more positive and hedonic attitude becoming more tolerant and exploring the pleasures and satisfactions that were denied.

Hopefulness and desire improve the *substantia nigra*. [80,85] And lacking scientific evidence, I invoke the vitalist

---

* *Grau, teurer Freund, ist alle Theorie. Und grün des Lebens goldner Baum* ("Faust", Goethe).

† Faustus dares to live (*Vivere aude*) against Horatio (*Sapere aude*). It is the dilemma of Genesis: the tree of Life is opposed to the forbidden tree of Knowledge. And Adam and Eve chose the opposite of Faustus.

Stevenson[218] who recommends late-life loves to combat the *petrifying action of the years*.

PASSIONS AS THE YEARS GO BY

Late-life loves are the most passionate. As the years go by, we toughen, we petrify. And Stevenson discovered that falling in love avoids the tendency to become fossils.

> *This simple accident of falling in love is as convenient as it is astonishing. It stops the petrifying action of the years, refutes cold and cynical conclusions, and awakens dormant sensitivities.*[218]

When you fall in love, your dormant sensibilities awaken. *Love moves the sun and the planets*, according to Dante. Freud explained that love (sex, pleasure) is the basis of motivation, the great source of dopamine. Sex (and more if love goes with it) is the best dopamine agonist, without the contraindications of ropinirole or pramipexole.

DIRTY OLD MEN DON'T GET PARKINSON'S DISEASE [79]

Freud scandalized society by discovering that children thought about sex, but it so happens that old people do too, and much more than you might think. At what age do passions fade? When do the eyes get bored of stalking adolescent thighs? Before he was fifty, Horace had forgotten those loves: *Put away this passion for the immature grape.* [107]

Lust for *unripe grapes* stimulates dopamine. I neither defend it nor censor it. I only write what I have seen: few parkinsonian patients were dirty old men... before medication. [79]

After taking dopamine agonists, the opposite happens: the patient has excess of libido, hypersexuality, but with difficulty in completing the action (he feels *more heat on the attic than in the basement*). Dopamine awakens the appetite, and its excess promotes addictions (pathological gambling, impulse control disorders).

THE PLEASURE MACHINE OF THE CRAZY PSYCHIATRIST

Wilhem Reich wrote a book (*The function of orgasm*[194]) and invented the *orgone* accumulator, a machine to unblock repressed sexual energy and thus cure neurotics. The madhouse was his destiny, but he ended up in prison, two places where many geniuses are sent. Madmen and geniuses share creativity, that explosion of dopamine, sometimes excessive or misunderstood.

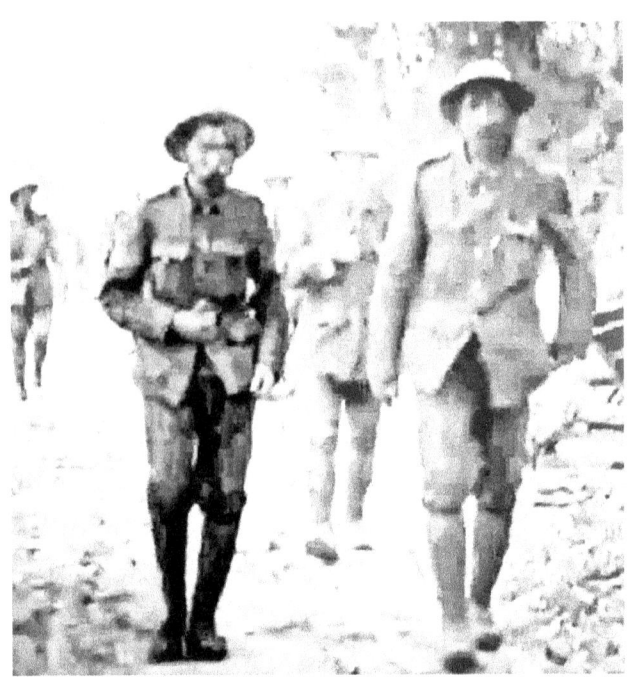

FIGURE 5. Stress causes Parkinson's disease. You will be convinced by seeing how prisoners of war walk and tremble in the films provided by Dr AJ Lees.

5. Stress kills neurons

Dopamine rises with pleasure but falls with stress, which kills the neurons where the neurotransmitter is generated. Dopaminergic circuits in the brainstem degenerate under chronic stress* [56,214,215]. In susceptible individuals, it causes anxiety and fear that precede motor symptoms.[45,46,188]

Stress influences the onset and development of Parkinson's disease. To ameliorate the symptoms and slow the progression of the disease, it is essential to avoid personal, familial, and social stress.

PSYCHOGENIC OR STRESS PARKINSONISM

Watch the Dr. Lees videos with prisoners of war[46,72], notice how these unfortunate men shake and walk, and you will be convinced that stress causes parkinsonism. I don't understand neurologists who still won't admit it.

The genome of Parkinson's patients is predisposed to the disease but is modified by the ambiome (environmental factors) as explained by epigenetics.

In susceptible people the disease is triggered and develops by stress and anxiety, and by toxic and other factors unknown to us. Scientists confirm that stress kills dopaminergic neurons.

---

* Estres induces degeneration of nerve networks in the initial segment of the substantia nigra, which regulate emotions and the stress response.[188]

Scientists confirm that stress kills dopaminergic neurons[46,104,188,215] and all agree that it worsens symptoms: tremor and blocking increase when discussing with a spouse or receiving bad news.

This is well known by the patients and their relatives, just ask them.

MISMANAGING PROBLEMS

More important than what happens to us is a matter of how we manage it, how we digest it. People with Parkinson's disease process adversity poorly, they become more stressed and internalise negative feelings.

The stress response* is highly dependent on the early stages of life. Initial experiences (maternal care is critical) cause definitive hormonal and cellular reshaping in the hippocampus, amygdala, and other limbic areas, reconfiguring cholinergic, dopaminergic and serotonergic circuits.

This early moulding or *forging* of neurotransmitters and neural networks will determine how adults will react to stress, their tendency to addictions, their emotional intelligence, and cognitive abilities.

---

* Stress response depends on the hypothalamic-pituitary-adrenal axis. Excess corticosteroid by stress destroys nerve endings in the striatum and nigrostriatal circuits.[214,215]

STRICT TEACHER, DEMANDING BOSS, NAGGING SPOUSE

Punishment in childhood[37], demands at work or reproach at home are stressors that kill neurons in the *substantia nigra*.

Anxiety is a disproportionate response to stress. One in three parkinsonian is depressed, and these are the ones whose motor and cognitive abilities deteriorate the fastest. A psychiatrist may be needed to resolve anxiety and depression.

The psychotherapist has a lot of work to do: childhood traumas must be forgotten, demanding jobs must be avoided, and no one should be allowed to reprimand you, reproach contaminates any relationship.

ANTICIPATORY ANXIETY

A version of episodic stress is the anticipatory behaviour, which is so common in the disease: they get nervous and apprehensive about what is going to happen or simply if they must wait a few minutes longer than expected.

When they tell the neurologist that they have worsened, it is a mistake to increase the antiparkinsonian drugs. A mild anxiolytic or, preferably, psychotherapy and natural sedatives (valerian, passionflower) are more effective.

*I WRITE WHAT I SAW**

I have become convinced that stress favours Parkinson's because of what I have seen and heard during 30 years as a neurologist, when I asked the third of the Hippocratic questions: what did they attribute the symptoms?

The businessman attributed it to the ruin of the business, the wife to her husband's infidelity. Others related it to the death of their mother or child, to disputes over an inheritance, to a demanding boss who persecutes him or to his wife who is a nagging machine. Also pending lawsuits, an abusive husband, sexual guilt or fear of hell are stressful events to which patients attribute their symptoms.

CLASSICAL NEUROLOGISTS AND JUDGES BLAME STRESS

Nineteenth-century neurologists also perceived stress as a cause of disease. Among James Parkinson's six cases,[168] an English sailor imprisoned by Spaniards blamed his sufferings in prison.

Charcot attributed his patient's tremor to being in danger of shipwreck.[29] Another French neurologist, Denombré,[43] describes the death of a child or husband, or a kidnapping, or a bombing, as examples of stress being the cause, and leaves this beautiful description:

> *Vivid emotions, violent shocks of mood, unheeded grief, great and sudden fear, have an unquestionable influence on the*

---

* The phrase is Quevedo's: *I write what I saw, I give to read my* eyes[184].

development of paralysis agitans, and observations to prove this are not rare.

In recent times, the tribunals recognise stress-related Parkinson's disease in their sentences about the son of a man killed by ETA (Audiencia Nacional) and a policeman (Tribunal Superior de Justicia de Valencia).*

THE DANGER OF SUPPRESSING EMOTIONS

Mark is PhD in Psychology and one of the patients I learned the most from. In his book *In search of my lost anger*[109] he relates how his illness began in childhood, when his emotions were suppressed by a strict edu-cation, and continued as an adult due to a very deman-ding job.

This connection of Parkinson's disease with emotional repression, where instincts are pruned, is also described by one of Dr Denombré's patients:†

My only fault has been that it's not easy for me to get angry.

Therefore, if repressing anger favours the disease, the treatment will be the opposite: not to remain silent, not to hide the injustice suffered, to bring it out, to shout it out if necessary: let the instincts express themselves with all their power.

---

* Audiencia Nacional (Sala de lo Penal, Sentencia 29/07, Madrid 2007, 14 May) and Tribunal Superior Justicia Valencia (Sala Contencioso-Administrativo 2, Sentencia 356/2020, 25 May).

† It is an interesting little book, *De la maladie de Parkinson*, Dr. Denombré (1890), which I translated from the French.[43]

PARKINSON'S AS A CULTURAL DISEASE

Neither animals nor savage humans suffer from Parkinson's disease. It is only observed in civilised people, and more in those who are very conventional and hyperadapted to social norms.

Some consider Parkinson's as a cultural disease[83], a product of the *graft* that civilisation has made on the animal we were: *Cultural animal*[167] is a concept of the philosopher Carlos Paris, and I was lucky enough to hear it live.

Gracián[89] praises civilised society: *Each individual is born a barbarian and is saved from being a beast by acquiring culture.* Culture has obvious advantages, but it requires the repression of instincts and emotions, the emergence of guilt and stress which worsen the symptoms and evolution of Parkinson's disease.

In animals and savage peoples this does not exist: there are no culprits in the jungle, guilt is an invention of society, a consequence of the transgression of a cultural ruling principle, as explained by the psychiatrist Castilla del Pino.[25]

SOCIETY AS A COLLECTIVE NEUROSIS

"Civilization and its discontent" (*Unbehagen in der Kultur 1930*)" reflects Freud's pessimistic view[69] on the cultural tendency to dominate instincts and suppress pleasure*.

---

* Controlling instincts reduces suffering, but also pleasure, because satisfying a domesticated instinct produces less enjoyment than that of an unrestrained impulse.

He compares the psychic evolution of the individual with that of society and culture.* In both cases there is a parallel between the repression of instincts and neurosis, in a similar way in the individual and in many *neurotised* societies under cultural pressures.

Emotional hygiene (so important for the Parkinson's patient) may consist of *undressing a bit of culture*, escaping from the social network, freeing some of the repressed instinct; I sense that it would benefit the patients, who are so socially hyperadapted.

GET OUT OF THE HERD, ESCAPE THE SOCIAL NETWORK

Let's look at some examples of (avoidable) socio-familial stress: family members celebrate Christmas meal and spend it worse together than alone. Why do you go to a meeting with neighbours, relatives, or work colleagues if you don't like them? Why do you have dinner with that married couple who envy you or with whom you don't sympathise? These situations will worsen your symptoms and, in the long run, the disease.

Seek people's approval and you will be their prisoner (Lao Tse). Learn to redefine the links with your envi-ronment, escape from the social network.

The greatest trick is to know wich cards to throw away (Gracián *dixit*)[89]. Get rid of bad cards... and of negative or unfortunate people. Get together with good friends, with

---

* *Culture* are productions and institutions that distance our lives from those of our animal ancestors to protect humans against nature and to regulate the relations between them[69].

what you enjoy and what they enrich you. Join the merry people and flee from the unhappy: *Et colle felices, miseros fuge* (in words of Lucan[136]).

COURT CONTEMPT AND HAMLET PRAISE[93]

Those who live in cities suffer more anxiety and mental problems than those in towns. Guevara's topic of withdrawing from social life (the court) and returning to simple surroundings (the village)* is continued in Fray Luis de León with his praise of the *retired life*, and others: *Let others deal with government, with the world and its monarchies affairs* (Góngora)[77].

Acoustic noise, and social noise, contaminate our cities. *What a restful life is that of the one who flees from the worldly noise!* (Fray Luis de León).[67]

In these noisy times, silence is a privilege. Remaining silent for several minutes lowers blood pressure and heart and respiratory rate, and decreases cortisol levels (stress hormone).[14,172,230] Silence regenerates neurons in the hippocampus and other brain areas relevant for memory, emotions, and motor skills: all advantages for the patients.

THE CIMARRON BROKE HIS CHAINS

Instincts are the brain's lifeblood, its best nutrient. The civilised world tames the *dormant beast* living inside all

---

* The hamlet is the ideal place for leisure and provides enough time to enjoy pleasurable activities without worrying about appearances; its food is fresh and there is no need for doctors because nobody gets sick (Antonio de Guevara, 1539).[93]

of us. Culture aims to control our natural impulses, and because of restraining instincts, the animal-turned-citizen is too weakened.

A *cimarron* is the one who has broken his chains, be it man, animal, or plant. I have seen its opposite in many fearful, domesticated, excessively educated Parkinson's patients. They are dutiful, highly cultured *urbanites* who have internalised rules and controls: the *tamed* male or female. Once in a while, try being naughty and a bit wild: it boosts dopamine.

THE POWER OF INSTINCT

Instinct* is lifeblood for the brain. We emphasize reading or solving crosswords to increase memory. But *Books are sarcophagi if they are not applied to the life* (Nietzsche).

Brain's strength lies in instincts. For higher cognitive functions to develop, cerebral cortex needs the energy of experiences and drives from the lower, reptilian brain. This is consistent with many of Freud's theories.† "The *Id* knows more than the *Ego* "[216].

Current neuropsychoanalysis postulates that our subjective identity, our *selfhood,* or *nuclear self* resides in

---

* Instinct (from *instinctus:* impulse, motivation) is a complex of external, hereditary reactions, adapted to a genetically unconscious purpose, expression of innate biological factors.

† Freud used the term *Trieb,* mistranslated as *instinct* (biological and innate) and actually it is *drive*, meta-instinctive, modified by psychic experience and exclusive to humans.

ancient subcortical neuropsychic processes that express affectively intense but non-conscious forms of experience,[216] and are discharged as instinctual actions outward or inward, in midline cortico-limbic circuits that are activated in REM sleep.[1,216]

PSYCHOTHERAPY TO MANAGE STRESS

To combat Parkinson's disease, it is essential to reduce stress, be it with psychotherapy, natural sedatives or even anxiolytics: this will be more effective than increasing Sinemet or agonists.

Psychotherapy is a pillar of the ecological treatment of Parkinson's disease. The patient will learn to reduce stress, to locate and reduce stress triggers, to relax, to reduce feelings of guilt and *ruminative* thinking, and to avoid social or family reproaches.

You will achieve a more hedonistic, positive outlook, you will enjoy life. With emotional hygiene you will forget hostile ideas or inflexible attitudes. Intolerance harms you and good humour is part of your treatment. Psychotherapy improves symptoms and the course of the disease and reduces the use of harmful drugs.

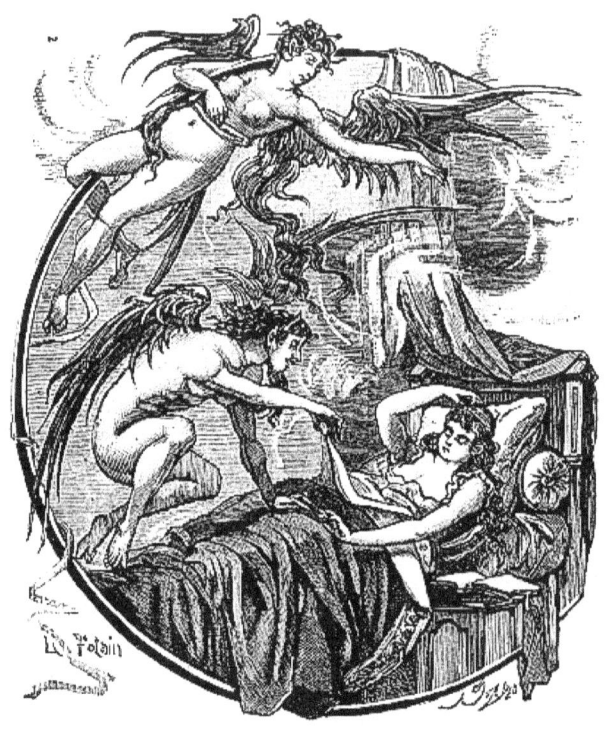

FIGURE 6: Dreams predict the course of Parkinson's disease. Sleeping unwell, or with nightmares or crying out is a bad omen, which can be ameliorated by reducing medication.

6. Tell me your dreams and I'll predict your future

The dreams of Parkinson's sufferers prophesy the future... of their disease. The content of the dream tells us how the symptoms will evolve.

Nightmares or dreams with screaming or violent content are a bad omen. On the contrary, restorative sleep enhances mobility, elevates mood, reduces the need for pills and improves the long-term prognosis.

Don't let drugs spoil your dreams.

*LIFE IS A DREAM**

The newborn sleeps and dreams most of the time. Sensations from the outside world bombard his brain, which grows, matures, and accumulates information from the natural and cultural environment.

Under the guidance of pleasure, it orients him to what is good for him, and with pain as a sentinel, it warns him of dangers. Little by little the child learns that he is not alone, that there are other beings closer (family) and more distant (friends and enemies), and that they are all governed by time, space, the sun... and social laws.

Neither of time nor of space there are limitations in dreams. Our true *self* emerges from sleep, our *selfhood* is

---

* *All life is a dream, and dreams are dreams*: Calderón de la Barca, "La vida es sueño" (1640).

in dreams. Sleeping and dreaming nourish our brain, develop neurons, and mature cognitive and motor capacities. We build ourselves according to the way we dream. Sleep and dreams are sources of physical and mental health, a treasure not to be missed. You should eliminate what keeps you awake or causes you nightmares. Start by supressing drugs that disturb it.

DREAM CONTENT PREDICTS DISEASE COURSE

How patients sleep and dream predicts how Parkinson's disease evolves. If you dream of strange animals, aggressive or distressing situations, you do worse than others. Very vivid dreams, which seem real, warn of hallucinations to come. Those who scream and punch in their sleep, as if fighting with their partner, are losing more neurons than expected, and this will affect them cognitively.

Symptoms will worsen if there are sleep disorders, and drugs favour them: insomnia, nightmares, REM sleep behaviour disorders[144], somniloquy, sleepwalking, daytime sleepiness, sleep attacks, narcolepsy, cataplexy, sleep paralysis, hypnagogic or hypnopompic hallucinations....

HYPNOS *IS THE* NIX *SON AND THE* ONYROS *FATHER*

Many religions consider dreams as gods' messengers. Dreaming is a *religion* of the mind[139] in the sense that it *re-links*, connects, in complex relationships, real, current events and emotions with ancient childhood memories or inherited archetypes. In dreams, emotional experiences are *digested*, psychically transformed, and the principles of reality and desire are brought closer together.

In Greek mythology, it all fits together: Night (*Nix*) is the mother of *Hypnos* (Sleep) who, in union with *Pasithea* (Hallucinations) had a thousand children, the *Oniros* (*Dreams*).*

In Parkinson's disease all become disorganised: the night does not lead to sleep and hallucinations are mixed with distressing dreams and unconfessable fantasies. Good night's sleep must be regained to prevent the disease from progressing.

OLD PEOPLE DREAM LESS

The newborn sleeps 18 hours, mostly as active sleep (REM phase outline) and alternating periods of passive sleep (prelude to NREM). In the following months and with external stimuli, they mature towards the sleep-wake cycle. And this evolution (reflected in the EEG) goes in parallel with the myelination and development of the brain,[156] which continues in childhood and adolescence until the *mature* nictemereal cycle in adulthood.

With ageing, REM sleep (the main phase for dreaming) decreases[41,92,156]. The healthy old people's dreams are less vivid and narrated in shallow detail; there are fewer

---

* The main *Oniros* are three: *Morpheus* makes us dream of human forms, *Phobethor* ("Phobos" means fear) induces nightmares with animals, and *Fantasio* represents the places (rocks, plants and waters) where we can become disoriented.

nightmares, and more childhood and adolescent themes.[92] Parkinsonian patiens also dream less and remember it worse.[92,239,253]

NIGHTMARES BEFORE PARKINSON'S

Not everyone with unpleasant dreams will develop Parkinson's disease, but frequent nightmares (more than one a week) increase the risk fourfold over the next five years.[158] At time of diagnosis, one in four patients admits disturbing or distressing dreams.[124,158,159,166,181,211]

FURIOUS DREAMS AND ANIMAL AS PROTAGONISTS

If the patient was very peaceful during the day and appears aggressive in the dream, or if odd animals are the protagonists, motor and cognitive deterioration will be more rapid.[18,19,61,232] *Furious** dreams, with greater belligerance, anticipate REM sleep behavioural disorders.[20,61,159,166]

Very vivid dreams are harbingers of hallucinations to come, and these predict further cognitive impairment.[202] Such a situation is an emergency that requires prompt treatment, and some recommend starting early with antipsychotics.[73] The foremost is to withdrawal medications that worsens dreams (agonists and antidepressants).

---

* This *fury* is attributed to the *dopamine devil*, due to dysregulation of this neurotransmitter (Lees syndrome).

SLEEP HEALS AND NOURISHES THE BRAIN

The ancient Greeks knew that dreams are healthy. In the temples of Asclepius (Aesculapius, Medicine's god), Morpheus was invoked with baths, incense, music and chants that induced sleep.

Sleep nourishes the brain; anyone who has had little sleep or nightmares the next day concentrates poorly, has memory lapses, and moves clumsily. Conversely, restful sleep, with pleasant dreams, encourages and improves mental and physical performance.

This *sleep benefit* is crucial in Parkinson's disease: if you have slept enough, and dreamt sweetly, you wake up with a clear mind, shaking less and walking better: you will need fewer pills.[204]

IF THE BRAIN SLEEPS BADLY, IT DEGENERATES

Sleep is life, but insomnia, nightmares and REM sleep disorders kill neurons. A brain that sleeps poorly degenerates rapidly; and conversely, neurodegenerative diseases such as Parkinson's and Alzheimer's cause sleep disorders from the outset.[208]

Ecological management of Parkinson's disease requires good sleep and dreaming, and sometimes the solution is simple: remove the drugs that impair them.

DON'T LET PILLS ROB YOUR DREAMS

Memory, emotions and unconscious impulses are reorganised during REM sleep.* Many drugs, mainly agonists, suppress or disrupt REM[176] this impairs the next day's activities and damages the memory and the psyche.

In Parkinson's disease, sleep is poor† in quantity and quality, and it will be worse with pramipexole or ropirinol.[40,256] Don't let them steal your dreams.

Anticholinesterase drugs (rivastigmine, donepezil) are sometimes prescribed to parkinsonians, but they may increase nightmares,[39,92,121] and this is more harmful than beneficial. Benzodiazepines relieve anxiety or restless legs syndrome (clonazepam) but shorten the REM phase and cause daytime sleepiness. The benefit/harm ratio must be assessed.

Hypnotics induce sleep artificially, like a switch. In some periods, a short half life hypnotic (lormetazepam) is necessary, but they disrupt the natural sleep architecture, reducing REM and memory. Amitriptyline is effective in some young patients with anxiety and tremor on account of its anticholinergic effect. It should not be given to older people because it causes confusion, bizarre dreams, and memory lapses.

---

* REM sleep regulates emotional homeostasis by activating mesolimbic dopaminergic circuits involved in self-referral processes, memory and the motivational content of dreams.[1,176].

† Fewer hours of sleep that is inefficient (decreases REM and increases superficial NREM), with more awakenings and movements.[256]

SLEEP HYGIENE

Hygiene* is the set of rules that promote health and prevent illness. To sleep well, there are simple, natural rules that everyone knows but few apply: during the day, sunbathe (outdoor activities) and, before going to bed, reduce artificial light (no mobile phone or television screens). Avoid coffee or stimulants, do not study or work or tackle problems before going to bed.

The bedroom is only for sleeping. It is time to rest, dinner was frugal and more than two hours ago. The TV off, the mobile disconnected and far away; we head to the bedroom to sleep, and maybe sex, but nothing else. No reading, no going over bills, no pillow-talking. And we will fulfil that personal ritual we most like to go to bed with.

NO ALARM CLOCK TO REMEMBER DREAMS

The alarm clock rings loudly, abruptly interrupting our dreams, and we spring up to get washed, have a quick breakfast, and go to work. How antiquated, how unnatural! It spoils the brain, undermines our health, and makes us unhappy. It's better not to do that, it's better to lazy around for a while, trying to catch the dream that wants to escape.

---

* Hygiene comes from *Hygia*, a daughter of Aesculapius, Medicine god. She instructed on how prevent illness (fresh water, cleaning wounds, healthy food, fresh air). Her sister *Panacea* ("the all-purpose remedy"), was the pharmacist: she carried a bag full of remedies for all kinds of ailments.

When we are awakened from a beautiful dream, we feel that we have been robbed of an emotional treasure. Let's keep it. Remembering dreams (even the not-so-good ones) improves memory and is very healthy for the brain. And even better if we write down what we have dreamt.

SUNBATHE TO GET A GOOD NIGHT'S SLEEP

Primitive man clearly distinguished day from night, but civilisation has blurred this separation, with artificial lights that alter the rhythm of waking and sleeping.[20]

We all have a *clock* that keeps us awake during the day and that make us sleep at night, with a rhythm of approximately 24 hours.*

Too little sunshine alters sleep, circadian rhythm and mood.[4,20] To sleep well we need to have received daylight and our brains need to know that darkness is coming. That's nature, imitate it.

MELATONIN ADJUSTS THE CIRCADIAN CLOCK

To regulate wakefulness and sleep, the circadian rhythm, the key is melatonin. With three hours of sunlight your brain will produce melatonin and you will sleep well. It decreases with age, and you can also buy it in pharmacies.

---

* This circadian (*about one day*) clock is in the suprachiasmatic nucleus of the hypothalamus, and is activated by the daily alternation of sunlight and darkness at night.

Melatonin is not a hypnotic, it does not relieve anxiety or remove depression, but it adjusts the sleep-wake biological clock, is an antioxidant and improves mobility in parkinsonians.[132] You can take a supplement (2-6 milligrams, sometimes more), one to two hours before bedtime. It is very useful in combination with phototherapy.[65,66]

PHOTOTHERAPY TO RESTORE SLEEP RHYTHM

To restore the sleep-wake rhythm, an alternative is light therapy, using bright light.

Phototherapy is the therapeutic application of light. Light, or a lack of it, acts on the pineal, hypothalamus and pituitary glands. It affects mood, weight, skin and biochemical processes (vitamin D production and hormones secretion).

In patients, light synchronises circadian rhythms which, in turn, improves sleep, mood and alleviates depression, sleep and other symptoms.[5,65,66,170,235,241,242,243] Dopamine agonists disrupt patients' circadian rhythms; bright light improves them without the need for added sleep medication.[58]

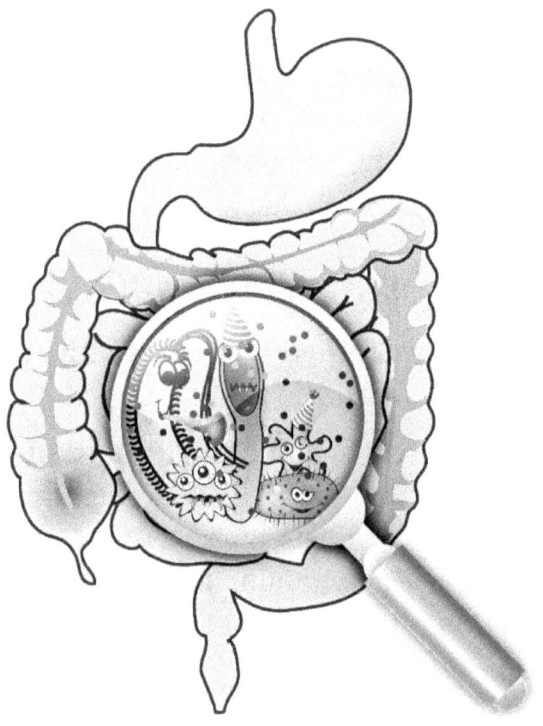

FIGURE 7. Parkinson's begins in the gut and depending on how it works, the disease will evolve better or worse. Intestinal function also depends on the microbiota (two kilos of bacteria that live there) and you have to take care of it with prebiotics (fibre-rich diet) and probiotics (yoghurt, kefir).

7. Parkinson's disease is born in the gut

If your neurologist doesn't ask you what you eat and how you defecate, change your doctor. Parkinson's pathology begins in the gut. That is where the disease enters and spreads. So, you must focus your treatment on the patient's gut. There we host billions of bacteria that digest food, facilitate the absorption of drugs, produce nutrients and neurotransmitters, enhance immunity and general health, and, especially, will be decisive for the progression of Parkinson's disease.

SLOWER THE GUT, THE WORSE THE SYMPTOMS

Many of the elderly are obsessed with bowel movements, with the intuition* that poor digestion is a sign of bad health... and they are right. Years before tremor or rigidity, patients are constipated and, later, the slower the bowel, the worse the symptoms become. Patients who defecate regularly have a better prognosis.

Many of the problems in Parkinson's arise from a malfunctioning gut, and there will be oscillations in response to drugs because they are poorly absorbed. Microbiota (those two kilos of bacteria we have in our gut) is altered from the beginning of the disease.

---

* Intuition is a shortcut to knowledge, it represents the intelligence of the subconscious (Jung), and it should be listened to...

PARKINSON'S DISEASE INVADES THE GUT

Parkinsonian pathology begins in the enteric nervous system, the so-called *gut brain*. First lesions coincide in time: in the olfactory bulb patients smell less), sympathetic ganglia (sweating, poor temperature regulation) and in the brainstem (sleep disorders).

According to Braak's hypothesis,[16,17,101,102] further expanded, bacterial flora troubles (dysbiosis) cause chronic inflammation of the intestinal mucosa and neuroinflammation that spreads through the microbiota-intestine-brain axis* . Other neurodegenerations (Alzheimer, Lewy's) would also use this intestinal gateway.[240]

MICROBIOTA, CONSTIPATION AND PARKINSON'S DISEASE

Constipated parkinsonian patients have different bacteria[15,70] and that dysbiosis influences the onset and progression of the disease.[70,105,261]

It is debated whether the lesions occur earlier in the brain, or in the intestinal mucosa, or whether the constipation precedes the microbiota alteration, or whether it is all at once. The fact is that they are related. That is why treatment of Parkinson's disease requires preventing constipation and taking care of the gut bacteria with dietary changes (prebiotics and probiotics).

---

* The intestinal barrier is breached, so toxic and inflammatory elements pass through this "functional hole" to the vagus nerve and into the blood, reaching the blood-brain barrier, which is also disrupted.[44,221]

MICROBIOTA, STRESS AND AGONISTS

Stress disrupts the microbiota and induces a proinflammatory environment favours parkinso-nism.[47] Bacterial flora is also damaged by antiparkinsonian drugs, mainly COMT inhibitors (entacapone, opicapone) and anticholinergics.[10] These microbiota perturbations will impair the progression of Parkinson's disease.

BACTERIA "COOK" WHAT WE EAT

We are what we eat and what our gut bacteria do with it. The microbiota cooks our food intake, processes it, and fabricates new molecules that will be passed on to the blood and brain.

Bacteria are the intermediary between our food and our neurons. We can eat healthily (Mediterranean diet, fruits, vitamins) but it will be of little use if our intestinal flora is deficient.

GUT IS A SOURCE OF DOPAMINE

Colonies of *good* bacteria protect us from Parkinson's and Alzheimer's diseases, and our metabolic and immune health depends on them.[219] Gut and microbiota *produce* dopamine (crucial for mobility and behaviour), plus other neurotransmitters (serotonin, noradrenaline, GABA) related to anxiety and depression.[48,78,219]

DYSKINESIAS FROM DIGESTIVE ORIGIN

Those who digest poorly have more dyskinesias. This may be due to the autonomic dysfunction of the disease itself, or to a bad microbiota that complicates digestion and slows down the intestine.

Drugs are not absorbed in the stomach but in the duodenum. If gastric emptying is delayed, levodopa is absorbed late and poorly, so its blood levels oscillate as do the symptoms: motor fluctuations or dyskinesias appear. Prokinetics (domperidone: Motilium) help, but the natural remedy is to improve diet and microbiota. Soya and other legumes decrease dyskinesias by increasing the absorption and efficacy of levodopa.[115,196]

LEVODOPA'S EFFICACY DEPENDS ON WHAT YOU EAT

With Sinemet you will improve a little or a lot depending on what you eat.[126]

In the protein redistribution diet, meat and fish are moved to dinner so that they do not compete with levodopa during the day. On the contrary, levodopa is better absorbed when mixed with carbohydrates (spaghetti, sugar) and in an acid medium. This is why, in an *"off" phase*, to ensure that the medication is absor-bed quickly, as a *rescue dose,* Sinemet or Madopar is crushed and some sugar and lemon juice are added. The effect will be much faster.

Levodopa absorption is also increased with caffeine and *Plantago ovata* seed, which allows levodopa to pass into the blood more smoothly, thereby with more stable and higher concentrations.[63]

DIET IS PART OF TREATMENT

With appropriate diet, nutrients and a good microbiota, the risk of Parkinson's disease decreases, and its progresssion is delayed.[249]

The Mediterranean[240] and fish-vegetarian diets[75,116,148] are very effective. Many other types of regimes have been proposed (hypo-caloric, carbohydrate-rich, etc.), which I detailed in another book.[84] Here I will focus on microbiota-enhancing (fibre, prebiotics, probiotics) to prevent intestinal inflammation and constipation.

Be careful to avoid toxic substances in food and in the environment. You think your salad is healthy, but if not washed properly, you could ingest the pesticides in tomatoes, the preservatives in canned corn, and the nanoparticles of petroleum left in your lettuce by the trucker's tailpipe. Industrial chemicals provoke Parkinson's disease.[26,42,74,115,152]

WITHDRAW DRUGS THAT CONSTIPATE YOU

First, negotiate with your doctor to withdraw constipating drugs, mainly agonists (ropinirole, pramipe-xole), anticholinergics (many antidepressants are) and opioid analgesics (codeine, tramadol).

Against constipation: a diet rich in vegetables and fruit, exercise and fibre supplements (*Plantago ovata* husks) with plenty of water (two litres), because they are not effective if not accompanied by sufficient fluids and can even worsen constipation.[6]

PREBIOTICS AND PROBIOTICS

Prebiotics are foods that we do not digest but which nourish gut bacteria and stimulate the growth of *beneficial* strains. They are a variety of fibre-rich carbohydrates, the best known of which inulin and fructo-oligosaccharides are found in some natural foods or added by the manufacturer.

Probiotics are live micro-organisms, bacteria or yeasts from food, medicines, or dietary supplements. Notably *Lactobacillus* and *Bifidobacterium* are available in tablet form, but we prefer those used to preserve food by fermenting cabbage (sauerkraut) or milk (yoghurt, kefir).

Probiotics preserve the microbiota, protect against Parkinson's and Alzheimer's diseases, increase metabolites and vitamins, eliminate pathogens, mature the immune system, and maintain the intestinal mucosal barrier intac[174]. Kefir is very effective against consti-pation in these patiens.[10]

EAT LITTLE, WALK A LOT, AND LIVE LONGER.

If they sold a drug to live longer and better, everyone would buy it. This panacea exists, it doesn't cost money and you don't have to go to the pharmacy either: *Less plate and more shoe* is the key to longevity. We have already seen this in *Rajoy's march*. Now let's talk about distancing the plates and not filling them so much.

Eating little makes yeasts, fruit flies, monkeys and humans live longer and makes them healthier and more resistant to neurodegenerative diseases, cardiovascular disease, cancer, and diabetes.[50] Limiting calories is the single most important factor that improves the signs of cellular ageing.[178]

The source of longevity is intermittent fasting. If you are fasting, your body uses up old fat reserves, and when you eat, it will accumulate new nutrients. Want to spoil a plant? irrigate it every day, and its roots will shrink; but if, occasionally, you leave it without water for a week, the roots will grow as they search for water.

BRIEF INTERMITTENT FASTING

Dietary restrictions reduce food or vary the frequency and intervals between meals. Their efficacy in preventing and treating Parkinson's disease is attributed to their effects on general metabolism, neuroendocrine, neuroinflammation and microbiome.[238]

During *brief intermittent fasting*, you do not reduce what you eat but increase the interval between meals. A short fast (8-12 hours) daily, every other day, or two or three days a week, etc. is all it takes.[50]

Intermittent fasting is more effective than nutritional supplements (which only act on one target)* . I recommend moderate intermittent fasting: two or three times a week, don't eat for 8-10 hours. This forces you to use up some of your reserves, which will be renewed, and regenerates bowel function.

---

* Intermittent fasting enhances hormesis, increases antioxidants and ketone bodies, promotes neurogenesis, and decreases excitotoxicity by up-regulating GABA.[155]

FAECAL TRANSPLANT AGAINST PARKINSON'S

To provoke parkinsonism in mice, we spoil their microbiota and then give them a toxin such as oral rotenone. But if they are first given a faecal transplant of bacteria that reinforces their microbiota, the inflammation of the mucosa is prevented and they are less affected by parkinsonism.[257] This protective effect of faecal transplants has also been demonstrated in mice inoculated with MPTP.[222,259]

Transplanting intestinal bacteria is already done in patients with severe microbiota problems, and in the future, it may be an option for Parkinson.ians with severe difficulties absorbing medication. It is a last resort, has risks and contraindications, and more relevant clinical trials will have to be awaited.

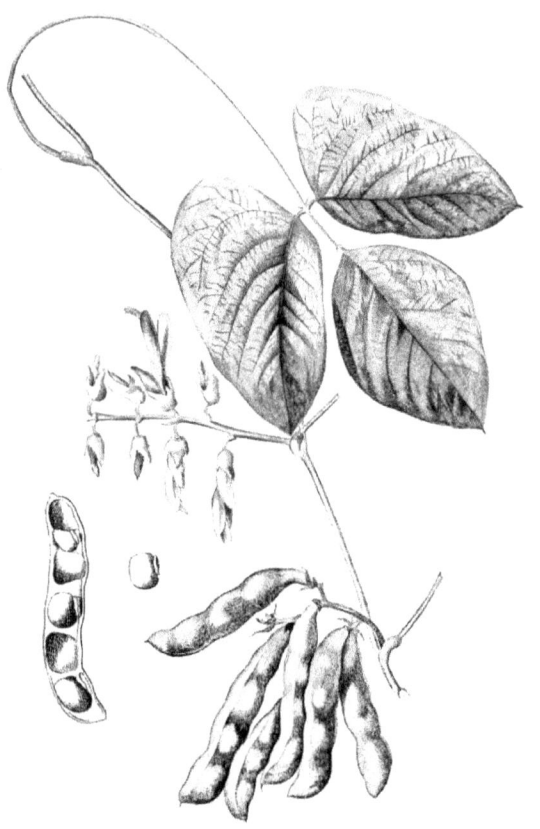

FIGURE 8. Natural levodopa is present in common beans. Mucuna is a bean that contains it in higher concentration because it grows in the tropics. It is the best natural product for treating Parkinson's disease.

8. Starting with natural levodopa (Mucuna)

In Amazonia I experienced mucuna myself and became very cheerful and enthusiastic, full of energy physically and mentally*. I had known about its properties since my 2014 book[81,82] and, one year later, I practised it on a patient in Manaus, with spectacular results (which I subsequently published in a journal and congress)[87,88.]

Mucuna pruriens is the best natural product for Parkinson's disease. There will come a time when you need levodopa, so you should look for a remedy in Nature rather than at the pharmacy. The broad beans (*Vicia faba*), that taste so good with cured ham, contain a small amount of levodopa. There is much more levodopa in the mucuna and that is why it improves Parkinsonian patients.

THEY DESPISE THE MUCUNA THEY DON'T KNOW

There are doctors who despise mucuna because they have not studied it. The most sceptical will recognise that common beans contain levodopa.† Mucuna is a

---

* The scientific part is in the journal and congress; I also made a video, reflecting this personal life experience: https://www.youtube.com/watch?v=PYYYT6Oezc3E&t=3s&ab_channel=NeurolologoGranada.

† Levodopa was discovered by Gugenheim after he ated too many broad beans (*Vicia fava*). In early-stage patients with few symptoms, broad beans would be a treatment option.[185,186]

bean which, because it grows in the tropics, has a higher concentration of levodopa.

Levodopa from mucuna is natural and has fewer side effects than synthetic levodopa from Sinemet, Sinemet Plus, Sinemet Retard, Madopar, Madopar Retard or Stalevo. These multiple preparations of synthetic levodopa are manufactured to suit different stages of the disease and different absorption profiles of patients.

Mucuna is just another way of administering levodopa, it is very beneficial for most patients, and produces fewer dyskinesias or complications. In addition, its effect is faster and longer-lasting, and it also improves mood: clinical trials show this and I have seen it in practice. Mucuna can interact with other drugs and should be monitored by a doctor.

SEED POWDER AND SEED EXTRACTS

The highest natural levodopa source is mucuna seeds, which also contain some serotonin and nicotine, and other ingredients only partially known. In Parkinson's disease, they are more effective and less toxic than synthetic preparations.[119]

Mucuna seed powder (as in Zandopa*) contains between 2.5 and 3.9% levodopa[119,190,233] meaning that about 30 grams of seeds are needed for 1 gram of levodopa (FIGURE 9). There are also various chemical extraction methods that achieve levodopa concentrations between 15-50%, even higher, for use in capsules or tinctures.

---

* Zandopa is the brand name of a standardised mucuna seed powder used in major clinical trials.

Two leading Parkinson's disease experts, Olanow and Lees, patented their own mucuna seed extract to treat neurological diseases and proposed it as an alternative to conventional levodopa formulations.[233]

MUCUNA IS BETTER THAN SINEMET OR MADOPAR

Comparisons are odious... for those who lose them.*
Patents on mucuna extracts and numerous clinical trials prove mucuna's advantages over Sinemet and Madopar:[34,35,119,233]

- It is less toxic than conventional levodopa.
- It is better absorbed, its effect starts earlier.
- Improves symptoms for a longer period.
- It does not require frequent dose increases to remain effective.
- It causes less dyskinesias, and even improves those†.

With these qualities, it cannot be denied that mucuna has a place in the treatment of Parkinson's disease. It is an additional way of administering levodopa that may

---

* The on time (motor improvement) and dyskinesias (complications) after 2 tablets of Sinemet Plus were compared against 15 and 30 grams of mucuna powder (Zandopa)... and mucuna won out.

† Mucuna generates fewer dyskinesias in patients.[35,119,233] In rats in which dyskinesias were induced, mucuna improves them, by synergy with its other ingredients.[96]

benefit certain patients at some stages of their evolution.

MUCUNA IS TOO EXPENSIVE WITHOUT CARBIDOPA

Mucuna does not contain carbidopa or benserazide. For this reason, to achieve the same effect as conventional drugs, the amount of natural levodopa to be administered must be multiplied by three or four times.[24] Since, in addition, the mucuna preparations sold on the Internet contain small amounts of levodopa, when administered alone, they have little, if any, impact on symptoms. Look at some examples:

To achieve the clinical effect of one tablet of Madopar or Sinemet, 1000 mg of mucuna levodopa must be given. That would be the same as 4 (7.5 gram) Zandopa cubes (in total, 30 grams of seed powder) (FIGURE 9). If capsules are chosen, this is equivalent to 20 capsules of the preparations that provide 50 mg per dose (such as Dopabean), and there are others that provide even less.

Imagine a newly diagnosed patient taking three tablets of Sinemet Plus 25/100* : that's 300 mg of levodopa, the same as 6 capsules of mucuna Dopabean (6x50 mg per capsule). But as Dopabean does not contain carbidopa or benserazide, for the patient to improve as much as with three Sinemet Plus tablets, the natural levodopa would need to be multiplied by 4; 24 capsules of Dopabean would be needed. This is why those taking mucuna improve almost by placebo effect (20 % on average).

---

* Sinemet Plus (25/100) contains 100 mg of levodopa, less than half that of a *plain* Sinemet (25/250 mg). What is *plus* is a higher carbidopa ratio (1:4 versus 1:10) to reduce adverse effects.

ZANDOPA IS THE CLINICAL TRIALS MUCUNA

The most valuable, scientifically rigorous clinical trials have been conducted with Zandopa, the brand name of a standardised powder of ground mucuna seeds. Not being an extract, its concentration (about 3.5 %) is lower than Dopabean or other capsules, and more powder must be given: it comes with a scoop for 7.5 grams equivalent to 250 mg of levodopa (5 capsules of Dopabean).

Since it doesn't contain carbidopa or benseracide, when given alone, 4 Zandopa tablets (30 grams = 1000 mg of natural levodopa) are needed for a clinical efficacy like that of one Sinemet 25/250, or almost 5 scoops when replacing 3 Sinemet Plus tablets (300 mg).*

GREEN TEA REINFORCES MUCUNA

Green tea potentiates the mucuna effectiveness because it contains substances with actions like those of carbidopa, entacapone and selegiline. This slightly increases the bioavailability and potency of natural levodopa.[87,88,134]

Doses must be considered, so after consulting your doctor, try combining mucuna with green tea in infusions or capsules.

---

* This happens with levodopa without carbidopa or benserazide (former Larodopa): the dose had to be increased a lot, with a lot of vomiting until Sinemet (from Latin: *sine emetere* = without vomiting).

ADDING CARBIDOPA TO MUCUNA

Carbidopa (and benseracide) makes the levodopa in Sinemet more effective by preventing discomfort (nausea, tachycardia) and does the same with the natural levodopa in mucuna. Mucuna with carbidopa greatly improves patients and even reduces dyskinesias.[187] Mucuna can also be combined with benserazide.[35]

Carbidopa is sold separately (Lodosyn) in the United States and Canada. If it is not available, you could take half a Sinemet Plus 25/100 (12.5 mg carbidopa)* and subtract the synthetic levodopa (50 mg) from the mucuna levodopa administered; note that, by potentiating it, you would have to reduce the dose.

What if you don't take Sinemet or Madopar? Then the mucuna is practically ineffective. Patients complain that it "doesn't do anything" and the reason is that decarboxylase removes it quickly from the blood, without time for a sufficient amount to reach the brain.

MUCUNA, SOYBEAN, ENTACAPONE, OPICAPONE, IMAO

The efficacy of levodopa from mucuna may be due to yet unidentified ingredients. A substance that acts as a natural COMT inhibitor (entacapone) has been found in mucuna; it increased the efficacy of levodopa in an animal trial.[169]

---

* With Madopar 50/200 the equivalent would be a quarter tablet (12.5 mg benserazide and only 50 mg conventional levodopa).

Soy inhibits COMT in a similar way to entacapone. When mixed (11 grams) with Sinemet Plus, rigidity improves for longer and dyskinesias are reduced.[151]

Atl the time of writing this book (January 2023) I cannot find any publication of mucuna combined with entacapone or opicapone. Nor have I seen any studies mixing mucuna with MAOIs (selegiline, rasagiline, safinamide). It is logical to think that just as they potentiate synthetic levodopa, they would do the same with the natural levodopa in mucuna. Let's wait further clinical trials*.

FRAUDS WHEN BUYING MUCUNA

Good and *bad* mucunas are sold on the Internet. If the formula content and concentration are not clear, do not buy them. In addition, many falsely advertise a quantity of levodopa that they do not contain..

I got the alarm from my colleague Tanya Denne (a researcher in Oregon) after analysing six mucuna products bought online[217]: three of the brands contained only 6, 34 or 40% of the levodopa claimed on the package. Three others had the levodopa they advertised and even more. The researchers do not cite the commercial names, but I was able to identify them from the data. I will not mention the deficient ones, but the brands I found to be compliant: Dopabean (Solaray), Mucuna Dopa (SourceNaturals) and Zandopa (Zandu).

---

* In plants there are substances with a similar effect to various antiparkinsonians:[189] something acts like safinamide in Banisteria [45] but is toxic; let them investigate.

In autumn 2022, another analysis[36] on 16 mucuna products showed huge variations in levodopa content: between 2 and 241 mg. If you buy mucuna, the package leaflet is not enough, request a certificate of contents differentiating the amount of powder or seed extract, the levodopa percentage and the actual content on each unit (sometimes they give the value of levodopa per 'dose' which may be two capsules).

MUCUNA UPDATES

On my website www.mucuna.es I provide additional information about mucuna.

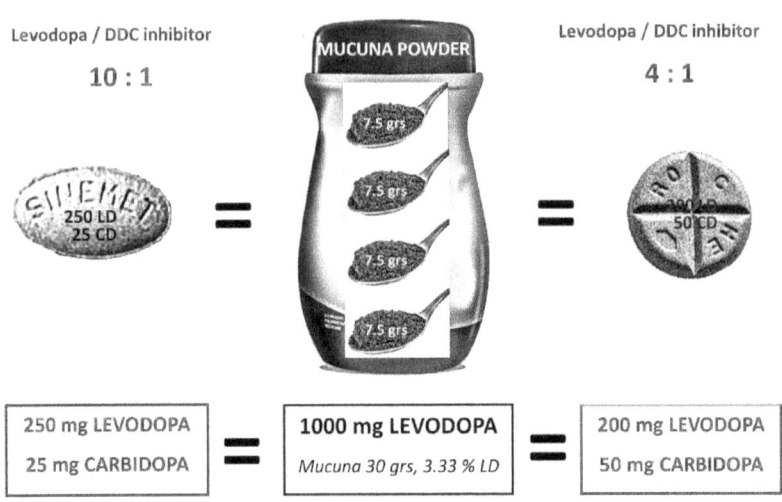

FIGURE 9. Adjusting mucuna doses is complicated. Lacking carbidopa, 1000 mg of natural levodopa (30 grams of seed powder) are needed to provide the equivalent clinical efficacy as one tablet of Sinemet.[88] Be careful if combining them because carbidopa in the tablet will potentiate the mucuna: consult your doctor.

9. Mucuna for medicated patients

A portion of conventional levodopa (Sinemet, Madopar) could be gradually replaced by mucuna under the guidance of a neurologist but should never be attempted by the patient.

As discussed in the preceding chapter, any levodopa (natural or synthetic) given alone requires four times the dose for the same clinical efficacy as carbidopa or benserazide. These greatly potentiate the mucuna, so it is necessary to know how to combine them.

In patients coming under general and antiparkinsonian treatments, the first step is to reduce or eliminate the less necessary ones. We will also check whether conventional levodopa preparations (Sinemet, Madopar) were being given adequately before starting to replace them with mucuna.

CHECK GENERAL MEDICATION

It is wise to go on a drug *discount*. Usually, as Parkinson's disease progresses, blood pressure decreases, and antiparkinsonian, antiprostatic, anxiolytic and cardiac arrhythmia drugs contribute to this.

I see patients who were once hypertensive but no longer are, while they are still on hypotensives and diuretics that they do not need. They are also prescribed prostate or heart medications, and they complain that they get dizzy with Sinemet... how can they not?

Limitations for the use of mucuna are the same as for levodopa but some mention that it may potentiate anti-platelet agents and should not be combined with anticoagulants. It has a slight hypoglycaemic and hypotensive action which should be considered.

RECONSIDERING AGONISTS IN THE ELDERLY

Mental changes and sleep problems often occur with dopaminergics or similar: rasagiline, rotigotine, amantadine, ropinirole, pramipexole....

This can occur with levodopa, but is much more frequent and serious with dopaminergics, which do little to improve the legs for how much they spoil the head, and much more so in the elderly. Dopaminergic agonists should be withdrawn or reduced after a certain age.

Conventional levodopa (Sinemet, Madopar) has a better benefit-to-harm ratio. It will continue to be needed but the aim is to gradually replace it with natural mucuna levodopa.

LEVODOPA "AD LIBITUM", TO ECONOMISE IT

A fixed schedule is recommended for taking the long half-life drugs (pramipexole, rasagiline, opicapone) and the delayed forms of levodopa (Sinemet Retard, Madopar HBS).

However, *fast-acting* levodopa (Sinemet Plus or Madopar) could be saved if given with some flexibility, occasionally changing schedules or dosage (within a range). This is nearly levodopa *ad libitum* (when neeedes, on demand).[100]

A patient suffering from dyskinesias *on* should not take the dose of levodopa scheduled for that time, and a patient *off* can bring forward the planned dose to a later time.

You may be able to accommodate the times and doses of rapid levodopa. Because some days you will need more than others, depending on how you have slept, weather conditions, joys or sorrows experienced, sport you have done, or the food you ate. In collaboration with your doctor, you may save some levodopa every day for months and years.

MUCUNA TO REPLACE SINEMET OR MADOPAR

Once general drugs and agonists have been reduced, and the conventional levodopa schedule has been restructured, it is time to replace some of it with natural mucuna.

We need a reliable mucuna, as many preparations do not contain the levodopa they are advertised to contain. I will give examples of two brands with proven concentrations: Zandopa and Dopabean (see previous chapter).

MUCUNA ALONE WOULD BE VERY EXPENSIVE

If a patient taking four tablets a day of Sinemet 25/250 or Madopar 50/200 wants to switch to mucuna alone, he would need 4000 mg of natural levodopa, i.e. 120 mg of seed powder (a whole bottle of Zandopa is 175 mg), or 66 capsules of Bonusan (60 mg) or 80 of Dopabean (50 mg).

This is affordable for few people in the Western world, with the paradox that in poor tropical countries, where

Sinemet cannot be bought, mucuna grows spontaneously, is very cheap and is an option there.*

MUCUNA USES THE CARBIDOPA OF SINEMET

Mucuna is four times more effective in the presence of carbidopa or benserazide. Therefore, patients who continue to take some Sinemet or Madopar while taking mucuna will save a lot of money because they will spend less of it.

That is essential to consider when adjusting doses. The problems are often greater when the patient who was taking only mucuna decides to add the conventional drugs may have an overreaction because the decarboxylase inhibitors will greatly potentiate the levodopa of mucuna.

CHECK THE INDIVIDUAL PROFILE FOR MUCUNA

Mucuna is another way of giving levodopa but not everyone reacts the same.

The first time a patient takes mucuna, I prefer to check his individual profile. Over several days, part of the conventional levodopa dose is replaced by the mucuna equivalent, or a little more (as the decarboxylase inhibitor ratio is lowered in the mix).

Subsequent changes will depend on the initial results; normally they will not be very evident if they are made at a low dose and slowly, but it is preferable to go pro-

---

* In poor tropical countries, the alternative is to roast mucuna seeds with results not inferior to conventional brands[24].

gresssively, so that later they can be increased. I give some examples as a guideline.

HOW TO REDUCE SINEMET PLUS 25/100 (yellow)

In a patient on Sinemet Plus (100 mg levodopa and 25 mg), one of these tablets can be exchanged for two capsules of Dopabean (each capsule contains 333 mg of mucuna at 15 % levodopa = 50 mg).

The effect may be a bit weaker, as the 100 milligrams of natural levodopa are devoid of carbidopa and therefore less effective... unless the effect of the previous dose of Sinemet still lasts.

Another option would be, instead of one tablet of Sinemet Plus, to give only half a tablet (50 mg levodopa and 12.5 mg carbidopa) together with a capsule of Dopabean (50 mg).

HOW TO REDUCE MADOPAR 50/200

The switching method is like that of Sinemet Plus, but taking into account that half a tablet of Sinemet Plus is equivalent to only a quarter of Madopar 50/200 (200 mg levodopa and 50 mg benserazide).

Thus, you can replace half a tablet of Madopar 50/200 (levodopa 100 mg, benserazide 25 mg) by two capsules of Dopabean (100 mg of levodopa). Or, to start even more slowly, take just one quarter Madopar (50 mg levodopa and 12.5 mg benserazide) combined with one capsule of Dopabean.

HOW TO REDUCE SINEMET 25/250 (blue)

This is a higher dose of conventional levodopa, 250 mg, which would have to be compensated with 5 capsules of Dopabean (only in this dose). This would still be insufficient because of the lack of carbidopa. It is therefore not surprising that attempts to switch to mucuna are sometimes disappointing.

I prefer a two-step changeover, adding extra carbidopa, as follows: instead of one tablet of Sinemet 25/250 mg I recommend taking one tablet of Sinemet Plus 25/100 (it provides the same amount of carbidopa as the whole tablet of Sinemet 25/250 mg) together with two capsules of Dopabean (100 mg natural levodopa). This makes an adequate ratio: 25 mg carbidopa for 200 mg levodopa (100 mg conventional and 100 mg natural). It is a good way to start this substitution process.

MANAGEMENT OF THOSE TAKING STALEVO

Here, in addition to conventional levodopa, there are two substances that change the metabolism of any levodopa: carbidopa and entacapone.

Entacapone inhibits another enzyme, COMT, which also increases the efficacy of the natural levodopa in mucuna. Together with carbidopa, the outcome is less predictable, but usually upward. Stalevo contains 200 mg entacapone in all combinations.

Stalevo 100 is equivalent to Sinemet Plus 25/100 with 200 mg entacapone: 100 mg levodopa together with 25 mg carbidopa and 200 mg entacapone. The simplest option is to replace one of the Stalevo 100 tablets with a

Stalevo 50 (50 mg levodopa with 12.5 mg carbidopa and 200 mg entacapone) together with a capsule of Dopa-bean (50 mg levodopa), making the replacement very similar.

DYSKINESIAS AND ADVANCED PATIENTS

For motor oscillations Olanow proposed frequent short draws of a levodopa solution.[157] This stabilises plasma levels, improves clinical response and reduces off and freezing.

Mucuna soon spoils in water (blackens) and should therefore be taken undiluted, but can be combined with shots of Sinemet Plus or Madopar solution, which is best preserved by adding a tablet of effervescent Vitamin C (for its antioxidant effect).

In advanced patients with dyskinesias, a rapid switch from pharmaceuticals to mucuna has been tried. They came with very high doses of conventional levodopa which were switched to quadruple doses of mucuna levodopa.[34] Clinical efficacy was similar, but half of the patients did not tolerate such a rapid change. This should be done gradually, or by combining carbidopa with mucuna.

MUCUNA CONTROLLED BY YOUR DOCTOR

Mucuna preparations vary widely in quality and composition. It is difficult to manage the doses of powder or extracts, their levodopa content, and the expected efficacy on symptoms.

It is risky to mix mucuna with Sinemet because carbidopa will increase its effects fourfold. Even more so if it is mixed without sufficient knowledge with Stalevo: the levodopa in mucuna will be potentiated by carbidopa and by entacapone.

Do not go it alone. Let your neurologist know the situation and he or she will advise you correctly.

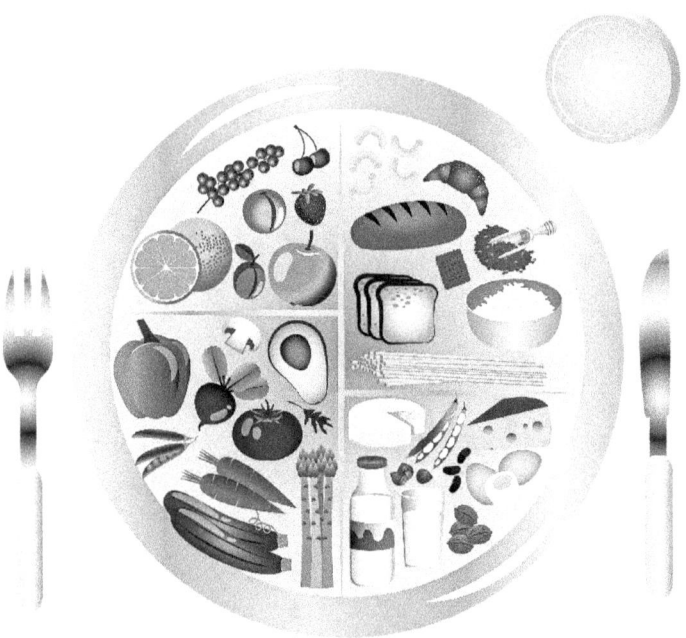

FIGURE 10. There are many important nutrients and supplements for people with Parkinson's disease. I describe the essential ones here.

10. Essential supplements

No single vitamin or nutrient has been shown to improve Parkinson's, but when some of them are missing, patients do poorly.

There are many supplements that are described in numerous well-informed publications.[141,142,146] I describe here only those that I consider essential.

B6 FOR THOSE TAKING CARBIDOPA

Carbidopa causes B6 deficiency which needs to be supplemented in those who take Sinemet (or Madopar's benserazide) for a long time.

Some people say that this vitamin is incompatible with levodopa, which, besides being exaggerated, is not true. Read the package leaflets carefully: B6 reduces the action of levodopa alone, but not if it is combined with carbidopa or benserazide (as in Sinemet and Madopar). On the other hand, carbidopa (and benserazide) causes a B6 deficiency which, if not compensated for, increases dyskinesias and causes peripheral neuropathy.

This neuropathy is very frequent and severe in those treated with Duodopa infusions (levodopa and carbidopa in large quantities), to the extent that B6 must be given preventively, and homocysteine levels must be controlled. Better if B1 is added.

B6, B9, B12 TO LOWER HOMOCYSTEINE

Homocysteine is high in the blood of Parkinsonian patients, and even in one in five of those newly diagnosed.[110] Levodopa raises homocysteine, and homocysteine deplete B6, B9 (folic) and B12, resulting in more cognitive impairment,[175,246] disease progression[162] and the risk of stroke.[95]

It is very easy to avoid all this: with a supplementation of B6, B12 and folic acid, at moderate doses.[95,220,252]

VITAMIN D DEFICIENCY IN THE ELDERLY AND PARKINSONIANS

Most elderly people lack vitamin D, and when they have cognitive deficits will improve if they receive it.[108,129]

Vitamin D has many important functions: it is neurotrophic, antioxidant, anti-inflammatory, and enhances cognition and the immune system.[30] Those with low levels are more likely to be admitted to hospital,[13] and during the Covid pandemic suffered the most and gravest infections.[90,145,173]

In Parkinson's patients, vitamin D deficiency is higher[11,212,258,260] and replenishing it serves as a preventive measure; although it does not ameliorate mobility, it reduces non-motor symptoms and has a positive influence on evolution: newly diagnosed patients with lower levels have a worse evolution in the following three years.[212]

It is a necessary supplement to delay the disease.

OMEGA 3 PREVENTS DYSKINESIAS

The health benefits of Omega-3 are well known. In *parkinsonian* monkeys, it relieves dyskinesias[201]. With a handful of walnuts a day and four sardines a week, you won't need omega-3 supplements.

GREEN TEA

Apart from its high antioxidant content, green tea contains substances with a similar effect to carbidopa and can be used to enhance mucuna (see that chapter).

KEFIR AND PREBIOTICS

As prebiotics, diets rich in fibre, and kefir as a natural pro-biotic are needed in patients with Parkinson's disease as we saw in chapter 7.

SLEEP SUPPLEMENTS

Restless legs syndrome may be due to iron deficiency. If plasma ferritin is low, iron supplementation may solve the problem.

Magnesium is another mineral with sedative properties that can facilitate sleep. It also improves constipation and cardiovascular health.

Passionflower, valerian and other natural sedatives are good options for insomnia.

CAFFEINE AND GINSENG AGAINST DAYTIME DROWSINESS

Coffee or caffeine supplements improve daytime sleepiness and relieve orthostatic hypotension (low blood pressure on standing).

Gingseng has a similar effect in keeping you awake and preventing pressure drops but should not be used in cases of hypertension or cardiac arrhythmias.

ROYAL JELLY AND PROPOLIS

Royal jelly from bees contains numerous vitamins and minerals, and no less than 578 amino acids, to which are attributed longevity and many other properties such as antioxidant, immunomodulatory and antiinflammatory.[2,143] Tests on parkinsonised animals have shown improvement with propolis.[76]

Beyond the trials, the surprising thing is that, with the same genes, a worker bee lives for 3 weeks and the queen for 4 years. The only difference is that the queen bee takes royal jelly. That's what convinces me, there must be something wonderful in royal jelly, even if scientists have not discovered it.

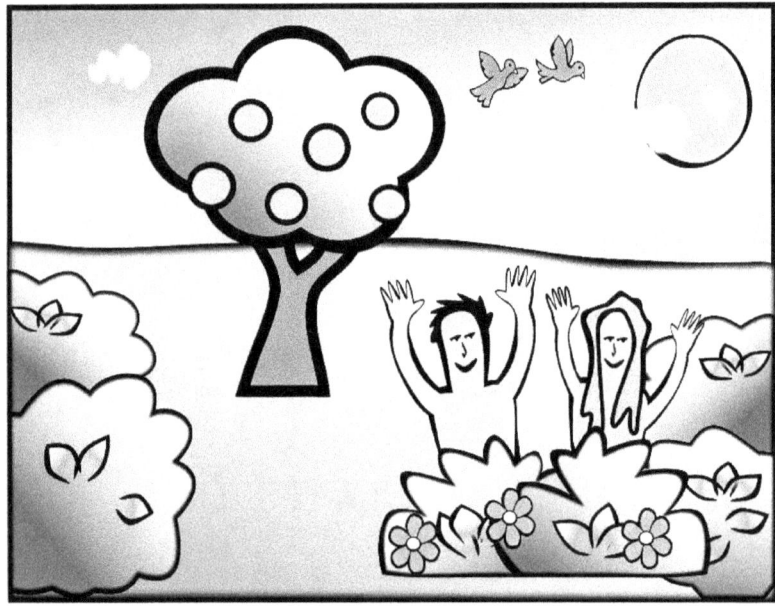

FIGURE 11: We need to get out of the pharmacy and closer into nature, to regain the power of instinct that nurtures the brain. We get sick the way we live and, conversely, we can regain our health by changing our lifestyle.

Epilogue

Parkinson's disease has developed in the civilised world, it does not exist in nature. It was not a threat to primitive man and nowadays we do not see it in animals or wild peoples.

There are genes that predispose to Parkinson's but they evolve in a *civilised* environment that has moved away from nature: toxins, social norms, technology, the artificial environment in which we live.

Man is already a *cultural animal*,[167] the cerebral cortex controls the reptilian brain, culture is a grafting of society onto the individual. This has advantages, but it restricts the emotions, suppresses the instincts that are the brain's lifeblood and separates us from the nature of which we are a part.

There is no treatment for Parkinson's disease in pharmacies, only to alleviate the symptoms, and in the long run the drugs pile up, with doctors increasing their number and dosage at each review. In a few years they cause complaints that James Parkinson never saw because in his time there was no levodopa, no agonists and no other supposedly innovative drugs.

Levodopa remains the most effective, has increased the quality of life and prolonged it; at some point it will have to be taken, but it is preferable to start with the natural one (mucuna). The other drugs may be necessary, but they have complications: often the diseases are made worse by the remedies. The drugs should be delayed and taken at the lowest possible dose.

There are only two treatments to halt Parkinson's disease: exercise and pleasure. The miracle key is exercise, physical activity in general and especially brisk walking, swimming, and intense training.

Pleasure, or rather pleasure-seeking, raises dopamine, and illusion enhances the *substantia nigra*; that includes avoiding stress: a demanding boss or a controlling spouse worsens symptoms and outcome.

Ecological treatment of Parkinson's disease includes all of these: exercise, pleasure, regulating sleep, taking care of the microbiota and diet (alimentary and also sensory), adding some supplements and, when levodopa is needed, starting with mucuna.

I will never tire of repeating it: we must move away from the pharmacy and get closer to nature, recover the strength of the instinct that boost the brain. We get sick the way we live and, conversely, we can regain our health by changing our lifestyle. Parkinson's sufferers who succeed to do so will live longer and much happier.

Bibliography

1. Alcaro A, Carta S. The "instinct" of imagination. A neuro-ethological approach to the evolution of the reflective mind and its application to psychotherapy. Front Hum Neurosci 2019; 12:522.

2. Ali AM, Kunugi H. Apitherapy for Parkinson's disease: A focus on the effects of propolis and royal jelly. Oxid Med Cell Longev 2020; 2020:1727142. doi: 10.1155/2020/1727142.

3. Ali NJ. Role of vitamin D in preventing of COVID-19 infection, progression and severity. Infect Public Health 2020; 13:1373-1380.

4. Amara AW, Chahine LM, Videnovic A. Treatment of sleep dysfunction in Parkinson's disease. Curr Treat Options Neurol 2017; 19:26.

5. Artemenko AR, Levin IaI. [The phototherapy of parkinsonism patients]. Zh Nevropatol Psikhiatr Im S S Korsakova 1996; 96:63-66

6. Ashraf W, Pfeiffer RF, Park F, Lof J, Quigley EM. Constipation in Parkinson's disease: objective assessment and response to psyllium. Movement disorders 1997; 12: 946-951.

7. Avery A. Aromatherapy and you. Blue Heron Hill Press, Kailua, HI 1992.

8. Avila A, Cardona X, Bello J et al. Impulse control disorders and punding in Parkinson's disease: the need for a structured interview. Neurology 2011; 26:166-172.

9. Baba Y, Futamura A, Kinno R et al. The relationship between the distinct ratios of benserazide and carbidopa to levodopa and motor complications in Parkinson's disease: A retrospective cohort study. J Neurol Sci 2022; 437:120263. doi: 10.1016.

10. Barichella M, Pacchetti C, Bolliri C, et al. Probiotics and prebiotic fiber for constipation associated with Parkinson disease: An RCT. Neurology. 2016; 87:1274-1280.

11. Behl T, Arora A, Singla RK, Sehgal A et al. Understanding the role of "sunshine vitamin D" in Parkinson's disease: A review. Front Pharmacol 2022; 13: 993033.

12. Berman MG, Jonides J, Kaplan S. The cognitive benefits of interacting with nature. Psychological Science 2008; 19:1207-1212.

13. Beirne A, McCarroll K, Walsh JB et al. Vitamin D and Hospital Admission in Older Adults: A Prospective Association. Nu-trients 2021; 13:616.

14. Bernardi L, Porta C, Sleight P. Cardiovascular, cerebrovascular, and respiratory changes induced by different types of music in musicians and non-musicians: the importance of silence, Heart 2006; 92: 445-452.

15. Bonnechère B, Amin N, van Duijn C. What are the key gut microbiota involved in neurological diseases? A systematic review. Int J Mol Sci 2022; 23:13665. doi: 10.3390/ijms232222213665.

16. Braak H, Del Tredici K, Rüb U et al. Staging of brain pathology related to sporadic Parkinson's disease. Neurobiol Aging 2003; 24:197-211.

17. Braak H, Rub U, Gai WP, Del Tredici K. Idiopathic Parkinson's disease: possible routes by which vulnerable neuronal types may be subject to neuroinvasion by an unknown pathogen. J Neural Transm (Vienna) 2003; 110:517-536.

18. Bugalho P, Ladeira F, Barbosa R, et al. Do dreams tell the future? Dream content as a predictor of cognitive deterioration in Parkinson's disease. J Sleep Res 2021; 30:e13163.

19. Bugalho P, Paiva T. Dream features in the early stages of Parkinson's disease. J Neural Transm (Vienna) 2011; 118:1613-1619.

20. Burns AC, Saxena R, Vetter C et al. Time spent in outdoor light is associated with mood, sleep, and circadian rhythm-related outcomes: A cross-sectional and longitudinal study in over 400,000 UK Biobank participants. J Affect Disord 2021; 295:347-352.

21. Calenda E, Weinstein S. Therapeutic massage. In: Weintraub MI (ed.) Alternative and complementary treatment in neurologic illness. Churchill Livingstone, New York 2001.

22. Cantor CR, Stern MB. Dopamine agonists and sleep in Parkinson's disease. Neurology 2002; 58(4 Suppl 1): S71-8.

23. Carroll LM, Morris ME, O'Connor WT, Clifford AM. Is aquatic therapy optimally prescribed for Parkinson's disease? A systematic review and meta-analysis. J Parkinsons Dis 2020; 10:59-76.

24. Cassani E, Cilia R, Laguna J et al. Mucuna pruriens for Parkinson's disease: Low-cost preparation method, laboratory measures and pharmacokinetics profile. J Neurol Sci 2016; 365:175-180.

25. Castilla del Pino C. La culpa. Alianza Editorial, Madrid 1991.

26. Caudle WM, Guillot TS, Lazo CR, Miller GW. Industrial toxicants and Parkinson's disease. Neurotoxicology 2012; 33:178-188.

27. Chahine LM, Daley J, Horn S, Duda JE, Colcher A, Hurtig H, Cantor C, Dahodwala N. Association between dopaminergic medications and nocturnal sleep in early-stage Parkinson's disease. Parkinsonism Relat Disord 2013; 19:859-863.

28. Chan ST, Tai CH, Wang LY et al. Influences of aerobic exercise on motor sequence learning and corticomotor excitability in people with Parkinson's disease. Neurorehabil Neural Repair 2023 Jan 12; 15459683221147006.

29. Charcot JM, Vulpian A. De la paralysie agitante, 1862. Spanish translation: González Maldonado R. De la paralysie agitante (bilingual edition). Amazon (Create Space), North Charleston 2013.

30. Charoenngam N, Holick MF. Immunologic effects of vitamin D on human health and disease. Nutrients 2020; 12:2097.

31. Chaudhuri KR, Pal S, Brefel-Courbon C. 'Sleep attacks' or 'unintended sleep episodes' occur with dopamine agonists: is this a class effect? Drug Saf 2002; 25:473-483.

32. Chen X, Liu F, Yan Z et al. Therapeutic effects of sensory input training on motor function rehabilitation after stroke. Medicine (Baltimore) 2018; 97: e13387.

33. Cicero (106 BC-43 BC, *Ad familiares* 9.4.

34. Cilia R, Laguna J, Pezzoli G. Daily intake of Mucuna pruriens in advanced Parkinson's disease: A 16-week, noninferiority, randomized, crossover, pilot study. Parkinsonism Relat Disord 2018; 49:60-66.

35. Cilia R, Laguna J, Cassani E et al. *Mucuna pruriens* in Parkinson disease: A double-blind, randomized, controlled, crossover study. Neurology 2017; 89:432-438.

36. Cohen PA, Ayula B, Katragunta K, Khan I. Levodopa content of Mucuna pruriens supplements in the NIH Dietary Supplement Label Database. JAMA Neurol 2022; 79:1085-1086.

37. Dallé E, Mabandla MV. Early life stress, depression and Parkinson's disease: a new approach. Mol Brain 2018; 11:18. Doi 10.1186/ s130 41- 018-0356-9

38. Darweesh SKL, Raphael KG, Brundin P et al. Parkinson Matters. J Parkinsons Dis 2018; 8:495-498.

39. Dautzenberg PLJ, Breuning L. [Rivastigmine as treatment for flashbacks and REM sleep problems in an older patient] [Article in Dutch] Tijdschr Psychiatr 2021; 63:70-73.

40. De Gennaro L, Lanteri O, Piras F et al. Dopaminergic system and dream recall: An MRI study in Parkinson's disease patients, Hum Brain Mapp 2016 Mar; 37:1136-1147.

41. Ontogenesis and organization of sleep] [Article in French]. Rev Prat 1989; 39:5-9.

42. De Miranda BR, Goldman SM, Miller GW et al. Preventing Parkinson's Disease: An Environmental Agenda. J Parkinsons Dis 2022; 12:45-68.

43. Denombré. De la maladie de Parkinson, 1890. Spanish translation: González Maldonado R, González Redondo R (eds). De la enfermedad de Parkinson. Amazon (Create Space), North Charleston, 2013.

44. de Theije CG, Wopereis H, Ramadan M et al. Altered gut microbiota and activity in a murine model of autism spectrum disorders. Brain Behav Immun 2014; 37:197-206.

45. Djamshidian A, Bernschneider-Reif S, Poewe W, Lees AJ. Banisteriopsis caapi, a forgotten potential therapy for Parkinson's disease? Mov Disord Clin Pract 2015; 3:19-26.

46. Djamshidian A, Lees AJ. Can stress trigger Parkinson's disease? J Neurol Neurosurg Psychiatry 2014; 85:878-881

47. Dodiya HB, Forsyth CB, Voigt RM, et al. Chronic stress-induced gut dysfunction exacerbates Parkinson's disease phenotype and pathology in a rotenone-induced mouse model of Parkinson's disease, Neurobiol Dis 2020; 135:104352.

48. Dohnalová L, Lundgren P, Carty JRE et al. A microbiome-dependent gut-brain pathway regulates motivation for exercise. Nature 2022 Dec 14. doi: 10.1038/s41586-022-05525-z.

49. Donoyama N, Suoh S, Ohkoshi N. Effectiveness of An-ma massage therapy in alleviating physical symptoms in out-patients with Parkinson's disease: a before-after study. Comple-ment Ther Clin Pract 2014; 20:251-261.

50. Dorling JL, Martin CK, Redman LM. Calorie restriction for enhanced longevity: The role of novel dietary strategies in the present obesogenic environment. Ageing Res Rev 2020; 64:101038.

51. d'Orsi G, Demaio V, Specchio LM. Pathological gambling plus hypersexuality in restless legs syndrome: a new case. Neurol Sci 2011; 32:707-709.

52. Dos Santos Delabary M, Passos Monteiro E, Gimenes Donida R et al. Can Samba and Forró brazilian rhythmic dance be more effective than walking in improving functional mobility and spatiotemporal gait parameters in patients with Parkinson's disease? BMC Neurol 2020; 20:305.

53. Dowd S, Vickers K, Krahn D. Exercise for depression: How to get patients moving. Current Psychiatry 2004; 3:10-20.

54. Edmonston D, Gruder O, Maitland CG. Whole Body Vibra-tion therapy with exercise enhances motor function and improves quality of life in Parkinson's disease. Archives of Physical Medicine and Rehabilitation 2016; 97: e74.

55. Edwards, L. Aromatherapy and essential oils. Healthy and Natural Journal 1994; Oct:134-137.

56. El Idrissi S, Fath N, Ibork H et al. Restraint stress exacerbates apoptosis in a 6-OHDA animal model of Parkinson's disease. Neurotox Res 2023 Jan 12. doi: 10.1007/s12640-022-00630-3.

57. Ellis T, Rochester L. Mobilizing Parkinson's Disease: The Future of Exercise, J Parkinsons Dis 2018; 8:S95-S100.

58. Endo T, Matsumura R, Tokuda IT et al. Bright light improves sleep in patients with Parkinson's disease: possible role of circadian restoration, Sci Rep 2020; 10:7982. doi: 10.1038/s41598-020-64645-6.

59. Evans AH, Katzenschlager R, Paviour D et al. Punding in Parkinson's disease: its relation to the dopamine dysregulation syndrome. Mov Disord 2004; 19:397-405.

60. Fang X, Han D, Cheng Q, et al. Association of levels of physical activity with risk of Parkinson disease: a systematic review and meta-analysis. *JAMA Netw Open.* 2018; 1: e182421.

61. Fantini ML, Corona A, Clerici S, Ferini-Strambi L. Aggressive dream content without daytime aggressiveness in REM sleep behavior disorder. Neurology 2005; 65:1010-1015.

62. Feng H, Li C, Liu J, Wang L et al. Virtual reality rehabilitation versus conventional physical therapy for improving balance and gait in Parkinson's disease patients: A randomized controlled trial. Med Sci Monit 2019; 25:4186-4192.

63. Fernandez-Martinez MN, Hernandez-Echevarria L, Sierra-Vega M et al. A randomised clinical trial to evaluate the effects of Plantago ovata husk in Parkinson patients: changes in levodopa pharmacokinetics and biochemical parameters. BMC Complement Altern Med 2014; 14:296.

64. Ferry P, Johnson M, Wallis P. Use of complementary therapies and non-prescribed medication in patients with Parkinson's disease. Postgrad Med J 2002; 78:612-614.

65. Fifel K, Videnovic A. Chronotherapies for Parkinson's disease. Prog Neurobiol 2019; 174:16-27.

66. Fifel K, Videnovic A. Light therapy in Parkinson's disease: towards mechanism-based protocols. Trends Neurosci 2018; 41:252-254.

67. Fray Luis de León. Ode I, Life withdrawn (1583).

68. Frazer M, Arcona S, Le L, Sasane R. Dopamine agonist monotherapy utilization in patients with Parkinson's disease. Clin Park Relat Disord 2022 Dec 17; 8:100173.

69. Freud S. El malestar en la cultura (1929). Alianza Editorial, Madrid 2010.

70. Fu SC, Shih LC, Wu PH, et al. Exploring the causal effect of constipation on Parkinson's disease through mediation analysis of Microbial Data. Front Cell Infect Microbiol 2022; 2:871710.

71. Gagliano-Jucá T, Li Z, Pencina KM et al. The stair climb power test as an efficacy outcome in randomized trials of function promoting therapies in older men. J Gerontol A Biol Sci Med Sci 2020; 75:1167-1175.

72. Gibberd FB, Simmonds, JP. Neurological disease in ex-far-east prisoners of war. Lancet 1980; 2:135-137.

73. Goetz CG, Fan W, Leurgans S. Antipsychotic medication treatment for mild hallucinations in Parkinson's disease: Positive impact on long-term worsening. Mov Disord 2008; 23:1541-1545.

74. Goldman SM. Environmental toxins and Parkinson's disease. Annu Rev Pharmacol Toxicol 2014; 54:141-164.

75. Gómez-Pinilla F. Brainfoods: The effect of nutrients on brain function. Nature Reviews Neuroscience 2008; 9:568-578.

76. Gonçalves VC, Pinheiro DJLL, de la Rosa T et al. Propolis as a potential disease-modifying strategy in Parkinson's disease: cardioprotective and neuroprotective effects in the 6-OHDA rat model. Nutrients 2020; 12:1551. doi: 10.3390/nu12061551.

77. Góngora L. Ándeme yo caliente (1581).

78. González-Arancibia C, Urrutia-Piñones J, Illanes-González J et al. Do your gut microbes affect your brain dopamine? Psychopharmacology (Berl) 2019; 236:1611-1622.

79. González Maldonado R. Conjectures of a neurologist who listened to a thousand parkinsonians. Create Space (Amazon), North Charleston 2014.

80. González Maldonado R. El extraño caso del Dr. Parkinson (a new vision of an old disease). Grupo Editorial Universitario, Granada 1997. Reissue in Create Space (Amazon), North Charleston 2013.

81. González Maldonado R. Mucuna contra Parkinson. Create Space (Amazon), North Charleston 2014.

82. González Maldonado R. Mucuna versus Parkinson's disease. Create Space (Amazon), North Charleston 2014.

83. González Maldonado R. Parkinson's and stress. Create Space (Amazon), North Charleston 2013.

84. González Maldonado R. Natural remedies for Parkinson's disease. Create Space (Amazon), North Charleston 2017.

85. González Maldonado R. Foreword. In: Díaz Márquez C (ed). Challenging Parkinson's disease. Grupo Editorial Universitario, Granada 1998.

86. González Maldonado R. Heterodox treatments in Parkinson's disease. Create Space (Amazon), North Charleston 2013.

87. González-Maldonado R, González-Redondo R, Di Caudo C. Benefit of the combination of mucuna, green tea and levodopa/benseracide in Parkinson's disease. Rev Neurol 2016; 62:525-526.

88. González-Maldonado R, González-Redondo R, Di Caudo C. The clinical effects of mucuna and green tea in combination with levodopa-benserazide in advanced Parkinson's disease: Experience from a case report. International Parkinson and Movement Disorders Society, Berlin June 2016. Mov Disord 2016; 31 Suppl 2, pp. S639.

89. Gracián B: Oráculo manual y arte de prudencia, 1647. Blanco E (ed). Cátedra, Madrid 2021. English translation: Robbins J (ed). The pocket Oracle and art of prudence. Penguin Classics, England 2011.

90. Grant WB, Lahore H, McDonnell et al. Evidence that vitamin D supplementation could reduce risk of influenza and COVID-19 infections and deaths. Nutrients 2020; 12:988.

91. Griesbauer EM, Manley E, Wiener JM, Spiers HJ. London taxi drivers: A review of neurocognitive studies and an exploration of how they build their cognitive map of London. Hippocampus 2022; 32:3-20.

92. Guénolé F, Marcaggi G, Baleyte JM, Garma L. Le rêve au cours du vieillissement normal et pathologique. Psychol NeuroPsychiatr Vieil 2010; 8: 87-96.

93. Guevara A. Court contempt and village praise (1613).

94. Gulas E, Wysiadecki G, Strzelecki D et al. Can microbiology affect psychiatry? A link between gut microbiota and psychiatric disorders. Psychiatr Pol 2018; 52::1023-1039.

95. Guo G, Xu S, Cao LD, Wu QY. The effect of levodopa benserazide hydrochloride on homocysteinemia levels in patients with Parkinson's disease and treatment of hyperhomocysteinemia. Eur Rev Med Pharmacol Sci 2016; 20:2409-2412.

96. Guzman JC, Otalora CA, Caro P et al. Decrease of dyskinesias in a model of Paarkinson's disease in Wistar rats, mediated by the phytopharmaceutical *Mucuna pruriens*. Neurology Perspectives 2021; 1:56-65. https://doi.org/10.1016/j.neurop.2021.03.011

97. Hamer M, Chida Y. Physical activity and risk of neurodegenerative disease: A systematic review of prospective evidence. Psychological Medicine 2009; 39:3-11.

98. Hammond DC, Kabbani S. Neurohypnosis. In: Weintraub MI (ed) Alternative and complementary treatment in neurologic illness. Churchill Livingstone, New York 2001.

99. Harro CC, Shoemaker MJ, Coatney CM et al. Effects of Nordic walking exercise on gait, motor/non-motor symptoms, and serum brain-derived neurotrophic factor in individuals with Parkinson's disease. Front Rehabil Sci 2022; 3:1010097.

100. Hauser RA, LeWitt PA, Comella CL. On demand therapy for Parkinson's disease patients: Opportunities and choices. Postgrad Med 2021; 133:721-727.

101. Hawkes CH, Del Tredici K, Braak H. Parkinson's disease: a dual-hit hypothesis. Neuropathol Appl Neurobiol 2007; 33:599-614.

102. Hawkes CH, Del Tredici K, Braak H. Parkinson's disease: the dual hit theory revisited. Ann N Y Acad Sci 2009; 170:615-622.

103. Helgerud J, Thomsen SN, Hoff J. Maximal strength training in patients with Parkinson's disease: impact onefferent neural drive, force-generating capacity, and functional performance. J Appl Physiol 2020; 129:683-690.

104. Hemmerle AM, Herman JP, Seroogy KB. Stress, depression and Parkinson's disease. Exp Neurol 2012; 233:79-86.

105. Hill-Burns EM, Debelius JW, Morton JT et al. Parkinson's disease and Parkinson's disease medications have distinct signatures of the gut microbiome. Mov Disord 2017; 32:739-749

106. Hironishi M, Miwa H, Kondo T. [Benefit of L-DOPA-without-DCI (decarboxylase inhibitor) therapy on wearing-off phenomenon in advanced stages of Parkinson's disease patients]. No To Shinkei 2002; 54:127-132.

107. Horace. Odes II, 5.

108. Hu J, Jia J, Zhang Y et al. Effects of vitamin D3 supplementation on cognition and blood lipids: A 12-month randomised, double-blind, placebo-controlled trial. J Neurol Neurosurg Psychiatry 2018; 89: 1341-1347.

109. Hurni M. Parkinson: Die verlorene Wut: Beobachtungen und Überlegungen zu einem außergewöhnlichen Krankheits-Fall. GRIM Verlag 2013.

110. Ibrahimagic OC, Smajlovic D, Dostovic Z et al. Hyperhomocysteinemia and its treatment in patients with Parkinson's disease. Mater Sociomed 2016; 28:303-306.

111. Imbesi S, Corzani M. Multisensory cues for gait rehabilitation with smart glasses: methodology, design, and results of a preliminary pilot. Sensors (Basel) 2023; 23:874. doi: 10.3390/s23020874.

112. Iucksch DD, Siega J, Leveck GC et al. Improvement of balance, motor aspects, and activities of daily living in Parkinson's disease after a sequential multimodal aquatic- and land-based Intervention program. Rehabil Res Pract 2023 Jan 9; 2023:2762863. doi: 10.1155/2023/2762863.

113. Jin X, Wang L, Liu S et al. The Impact of mind-body exercises on motor function, depressive symptoms, and quality of life in Parkinson's disease: a systematic review and meta-analysis. Int J Environ Res Public Health 2019; 17:31.

114. Johansson ME, Cameron IGM, Van der Kolk NM et al. Aerobic exercise alters brain function and structure in Parkinson's Disease: a randomized controlled trial. Ann Neurol 2022; 91:203-216.

115. Jokanović M, Oleksak P, Kuca K. Multiple neurological effects associated with exposure to organophosphorus pesticides in man. Toxicology 2023; 484:153407.

116. Kang JH, Ascherio A, Groodstein F. Fruit and vegetable consumption and cognitive decline in aging women. Annals of Neurology 2005; 57:713-720.

117. Karbowniczek A, Niewiadomski W, Niewiadomska G. Impact of the whole body vibration training on the motor symptoms in Parkinson disease patients. Parkinsonism & Related Disorders 2016; 22, Supplement 2:e66-e67.

118. Karpodini CC, Dinas PC, Angelopoulou E et al. Rhythmic cueing, dance, resistance training, and Parkinson's disease: A systematic review and meta-analysis. Front Neurol 2022; 13:875178.

119. Katzenschlager R, Evans A, Manson A et al. *Mucuna pruriens* in Parkinson's disease: a double blind clinical and pharmacological study. J Neurol Neurosurg Psychiatry 2004; 75:1672-1677.

120. Katzenschlager R, Lees AJ. Treatment of Parkinson's disease: levodopa as the first choice. J Neurol 2002; 249 Suppl 2:II19-24.

121. Kitabayashi Y, Ueda H, Tsuchida H et al. Donepezil-induced nightmares in mild cognitive impairment. Psychiatry Clin Neurosci 2006; 60:123-124.

122. Koepp MJ, Gunn RN, Lawrence AD et al. Evidence for striatal dopamine release during a video game. Nature 1998; 393:266-268.

123. Kulisevsky J, Roldan E. Hallucinations and sleep disturbances in Parkinson's disease. Neurology 2004; 63(8 Suppl 3): S28-30.

124. Kumar S, Bhatia M, Behari M. Sleep disorders in Parkinson's disease. Mov Disord 2002; 17:775-781.

125. Kwok JJY, Choi KC, Chan HYL. Effects of mind-body exercises on the physiological and psychosocial well-being of individuals with Parkinson's disease: A systematic review and meta-analysis. Complement Ther Med 2016; 29:121-131.

126. Keun JTB, Arnoldussen IA, Vriend C, van de Rest O. Dietary approaches to improve efficacy and control side effects of levodopa therapy in Parkinson's disease: a systematic review. Adv Nutr 2021; 12:2265-2287.

127. LeBourgeois MK, Dean DC, Deoni SCL et al. A simple sleep EEG marker in childhood predicts brain myelin 3.5 years later. Neuroimage 2019; 199:342-350.

128. Lees AJ. Drugs for Parkinson's disease. J Neurol Neurosurg Psychiatry 2002; 73:607-610.

129. Lewis JE, Poles J, Shaw DP et al. The effects of twenty-one nutrients and phytonutrients on cognitive function: A narrative review. J Clin Transl Res 2021; 7:575-620.

130. Li BD, Bi ZY, Liu JF et al. Adverse effects produced by different drugs used in the treatment of Parkinson's disease: A mixed treatment comparison. CNS Neurosci Ther 2017; 23: 827-842.

131. Li BD, Cu JJ, Song J et al. Comparison of the efficacy of different drugs on non-motor symptoms of Parkinson's disease: a network meta-analysis. Cell Physiol Biochem 2018; 45:119-130.

132. Liguori C, Fernandes M, Cerroni R et al. Effects of melatonin prolongedrelease -on both sleep and motor symptoms in Parkinson's disease: a preliminary evidence. Neurol Sci 2022; 43:5355-5362.

133. Lima LO, Scianni A, Rodrigues-de-Paula F. Progressive resistance exercise improves strength and physical performance in people with mild to moderate Parkinson's disease: a systematic review. J Physiother 2013; 59:7-13.

134. Lin SJ, Tai L, Huang YJ et al. Effect of catechin and commercial preparation of green tea essence on the pharmacokinetics of l-dopa in rabbits. Biomed Chromatogr 2021; 35: e5227.

135. Lord S, Godfrey A, Galna B et al. Ambulatory activity in incident Parkinson's: more than meets the eye? J Neurol 2013; 260:2964-2972.

136. Lucan. Pharsalia, VIII, 487.

137. Maguire EA, Woollett K, Spiers HJ. London taxi drivers and bus drivers: a structural MRI and neuropsychological analysis. Hippocampus 2006; 16:1091-1101.

138. Mak MKY, Wong-Yu ISK. Six-month community-based community-based brisk wal-king and balance exercise alleviates motor symptoms and promotes functions in people with Parkinson's disease: A Randomized controlled trial. J Parkinsons Dis 2021; 11:1431-1441.

139. Mancia M. The dream as religion of the mind. Int J Psychoanal 1988; 69:419-426.

140. Manyam BV, Sanchez-Ramos JR. Traditional and complementary therapies in Parkinson's disease. Adv Neurol 1999; 80:565-574.

141. Márquez Rivera J. A different way of looking at Parkinson's disease. Create Space (Amazon) 2015.

142. Márquez Rivera J. The cure for Parkinson's disease. Create Space (Amazon) 2021.

143. Martínez-Chacón G, Paredes-Barquero M, YakhineYakhine-Diop SMS et al. Neuroprotective properties of queen bee acid by autophagy induction. Cell Biol Toxicol 2021 Aug 27. doi: 10.1007/s10565-021-09625-w. Online ahead of print.

144. McCarter SJ, St Louis EK, Boeve BF. REM sleep behavior disorder and REM sleep without atonia as an early manifestation of degenerative neurological disease. Curr Neurol Neurosci Rep 2012; 12:182-192.

145. Mercola J, Grant WB, Wagner CL. Evidence regarding vitamin D and risk of COVID-19 and its severity. Nutrients 2020; 12:3361.

146. Mischley LK. Natural therapies for Parkinson's disease. Coffeetown press, Seattle 2010.

147. Mitchell D. Promoting enjoyment and self-belief through work rehabilitation. Arch Psychiatr Nurs 1998; 12:344-50.

148. Morris MC, Evans DA, Tangney CC et al. Associations of vegetable and fruit consumption with age-related cognitive change. Neurology 2006; 67:1370-1376.

149. Müller-RebsteiMüller-Rebstein S, Trenkwalder C, Ebentheuer J et al. Drug safety analysis in a real-life cohort of Parkinson's disease patients with polypharmacy. CNS Drugs 2017; 31:1093-1102.

150. Murata M. Levodopa in the early treatment of Parkinson's disease. Parkinsonism Relat Disord 2009; 15 Suppl 1: S17-20.

151. Nagashima Y, Kondo T, Sakata M et al. Effects of soybean ingestion on pharmacokinetics of levodopa and motor symptoms of Parkinson's disease-in relation to the effects of *Mucuna pruriens*. J Neurol Sci 2016; 361:229-234.

152. Nandipati S, Litvan I et al. Environmental Exposures and Parkinson's Disease. Int J Environ Res Public Health 2016; 13:881.

153. Nascimento CMC, Ayan C, Cancela JM et a. Effect of a multimodal exercise program on sleep disturbances and instrumental activities of daily living performance on Parkinson's and Alzheimer's disease patients. Geriatr Gerontol Int 2014; 14:259-266.

154. Neagoe AD. Delirium with manic and psychotic features associated with amantadine. Gen Hosp Psychiatry 2013; 35:680.e7-8. doi: 10.1016.

155. Neth BJ, Bauer BA, Benarroch EE, Savica R. The role of intermittent fasting in Parkinson's disease. Front Neurol 2021; 12:682184.

156. Ohayon MC, Carskadon MA, Guilleminault C, Vitiello MV. Meta-analysis of quantitative sleep parameters from childhood to old age in healthy individuals: developing normative sleep values across the human lifespan. Sleep 2004; 27:1255-1273.

157. Olanow CW, Torti M, Kieburtz K et al. Continuous versus intermittent oral administration of levodopa in Parkinson's disease patients with motor fluctuations: A pharmacokinetics, safety, and efficacy study. Mov Disord 2019; 34:425-429.

158. Otaiku AI. Distressing dreams and risk of Parkinson's disease: A population-based cohort study. EClinicalMedicine 2022; 48:101474.

159. Otaiku AI. Dream content predicts motor and cognitive decline in Parkinson's disease. Mov Disord Clin Pract. 2021; 8:1041-1051.

160. Ottosson J, Lavesson L, Pinzke S, Grahn P. The significance of experiences of nature for people with Parkinson's disease, with special focus on freezing of gait-the necessity for a biophilic environment. A multi-method single subject study. Int J Environ Res Public Health 2015; 12: 7274-7299

161. Ouchi Y, Kanno T, Okada H et al. Changes in dopamine availability in the nigrostriatal and mesocortical dopaminergic systems by gait in Parkinson's disease. Brain 2001; 124:784-792.

162. Ozer F, Meral H, Hanoglu L et al. Plasma homocysteine levels in patients treated with levodopa: motor and cognitive associations. Neurol Res 2006; 28:853-858.

163. Pacchetti C, Aglieri R, Mancini F, Martignoni E, Nappi G. Active music therapy and Parkinson's disease: methods. Funct Neurol 1998; 13:57-67.

164. Pacchetti C, Mancini F, Aglieri R, Fundaro C, Martignoni E, Nappi G. Active music therapy in Parkinson's disease: an integrative method for motor and emotional rehabilitation. Psychosom Med 2000; 62: 386-393.

165. Pagano G, Tan EE, Haider JM, Bautista A, Tagliati M. Constipation is reduced by beta-blockers and increased by dopaminergic medications in Parkinson's disease. Parkinsonism Relat Disord 2015; 21:120-125.

166. Paiva T, Bugalho P, Bentes C. Dreaming and cognition in patients with frontotemporal dysfunction. Conscious Cogn 2011; 20:1027-1035.

167. Paris, C. The cultural animal. Barcelona : Crítica, 1994.

168. Parkinson J. An assay on the shaking palsy. Sherwood, Neely & Jones, London 1817. Spanish translation (bilingual edition): González Maldonado R, Morata Pérez J (eds). An essay on shaking palsy. Amazon (Create Space), North Charleston 2013.

169. Parrales-Macias V, Harfouche A, Ferrié L et al. Effects of a new natural catechol-O-methyl transferase inhibitor on two in vivo models of Parkinson's disease. ACS Chem Neurosci 2022; 13:3303-3313.

170. Paus S, et al. Bright light therapy in PD: a pilot study. Mov Di-sord 2007; 22:1495-1498.

171. Paus S, Brecht HM, Köster J et al. Sleep attacks, daytime sleepiness, and dopamine agonists in Parkinson's disease. Mov Disord 2003; 18:659-667.

172. Pfeifer E, Wittmann M. Waiting, thinking, and feeling: variations in the perception of time during silence. Front Psychol 2020; 11: 02. doi: 10.3389/fpsyg.2020.00602

173. Pereira M, Dantas A, Galvão LM et al. Vitamin D deficiency aggravates COVID-19: systematic review and meta-analysis, Nutr 2022; 62:1308-1316.

174. Pereira TMC, Côco LZ, Ton AMM et al. The emerging scenario of the gut-brain axis: the therapeutic actions of the new actor kefir against neurodegenerative diseases. Antioxidants (Basel) 2021; 10:1845.

175. Periñán MT, Macías-García D, Jesús S et al. Homocysteine levels, genetic background, and cognitive impairment in Parkinson's disease. J Neurol 2023; 270:477-485.

176. Perogamvros L, Schwartz S. The roles of the reward system in sleep and dreaming. Neurosci Biobehav Rev 2012; 36:1934-1951.

177. Phuenpathom W, Panyakaew P, Vateekul P et al. Vibratory and plantar pressure stimulation: Steps to improve freezing of gait in Parkinson's disease. Parkinsonism & Related Disorders. Available online 28 October 2022.

178. Picca A, Pesce V, Lezza AMS. Does eating less make you live longer and better? An update on calorie restriction. Clin Interv Aging 2017; 12:1887-1902.

179. Pluck GC, Brown RG. Apathy in Parkinson's disea-se. J Neurol Neurosurg Psychiatry 2002; 73:636-642.

180. Poewe W. When a Parkinson's disease patient starts to hallucinate. Pract Neurol 2008; 8:238-241.

181. Pont-Sunyer C, Hotter A, Gaig C, et al. The onset of nonmotor symptoms in Parkinson's disease (the ONSET PD study). Mov Disord 2015; 30:229-237.

182. Poortvliet PC, Gluch A, Silburn PA, Mellick GD. The Queensland Parkinson's Project: An overview of 20 years of mortality from Parkinson's disease. J Mov Disord 2021; 14:34-41.

183. Proust M. Du côté de chez Swann (À la recherche du temps perdu). Salinas P (Trad). Por el camino de Swann (In Search of Lost Time). Unidad Editorial, Madrid 1999.

184. Quevedo y Villegas F. Grandes anales de quince días, historias de muchos siglos que pasaron en un mes. Imprenta de Sancha, posthumous edition 1794.

185. Rabey JM, Vered Y, Shabtai H et al. Broad bean (*Vicia faba*) consumption and Parkinson's disease. Adv Neurol 1993; 60:681-684.

186. Rabey JM, Vered Y, Shabtai H et al. Improvement of parkinsonian features correlate with high plasma levodopa values after broad bean (*Vicia faba*) consumption. J Neurol Neurosurg Psychiatry 1992; 55:725-727.

187. Radder DLM, Groenestege ATT, Boers I et al. *Mucuna Pruriens* combined with carbidopa in Parkinson's disease: A case report. J Parkinsons Dis 2019; 9:437-439.

188. Radulovic J, Ivkovic S, Adzic M. From chronic stress and anxiety to neurodegeneration: focus on neuromodulation of the axon initial segment. Handbook of Clinical Neurology 2022; 184: 481-495.

189. Rai SN, Mishra D, Singh P et al. Therapeutic applications of mushrooms and their biomolecules along with a glimpse of *in silico* approach in neurodegenerative diseases. Biomedicine & Pharmacotherapy 2021; 137:111377

190. Raina AP, Khatri R. Quantitative determination of L-DOPA in seeds of *mucuna pruriens* germplasm by high performance thin layer chromatography. Indian J Pharm Scienc 2011; 73:459-462.

191. Raphael A. "Ahh! Aromatherapy." Delicious 1994; 12:47-48.

192. Rascol O, Brooks DJ, Korczyn AD, De Deyn PP, Clarke CE, Lang AE. A five-year study of the incidence of dyskinesia in patients with early Parkinson's disease who were treated with ropinirole or levodopa. N Engl J Med 2000; 342:1484-1491.

193. Rascol O, Brooks DJ, Korczyn AD et al. Development of dyskinesias in a 5-year trial of ropinirole and L-dopa. Mov Disord 2006; 21:1844-1850.

194. Reich W. The function of the orgasm. Orgone Institute Press, New York 1927. Translation: The function of the orgasm. Paidós, Buenos Aires 1974.

195. Reuter I, Engelhardt M, Stecker K, Baas H. Therapeutic value of exercise training in Parkinson's disease, Med Sci Sports Exerc 1999; 31:1544-1549.

196. Rijntjes M. Knowing your beans in Parkinson's disease: a critical assessment of current knowledge about different beans and their compounds in the treatment of Parkinson's disease and in animal models. Parkinsons Dis 2019; 2019:1349509.

197. Rochester L, Baker K, Hetherington V et al. Evidence for motor learning in Parkinson's disease: acquisition, automaticity and retention of cued gait performance after training with external rhythmical cues. Brain Res 2010; 1319:103-111.

198. Rong S, Xu G, Liu B et al. Trends in mortality from Parkinson disease in the United States, 1999-2019. Neurology 2021; 97: e1986-e1993.

199. Rosenfeldt AB, Koop MM, Penko AL, Alberts JL. Individuals with Parkinson disease are adherent to a high-intensity community-based cycling exercise program. J Neurol Phys Ther 2022; 46:73-80.

200. Rowe PL, Taflan S, Hahne AJ. Does the addition of whole-body vibration training improve postural stability and lower limb strength during rehabilitation following anterior cruciate ligament reconstruction: a systematic review with meta-analysis. Clin J Sport Med 2022; 32:627-634.

201. Samadi P, Grégoire L, Rouillard C et al. Docosahexaenoic acid reduces levodopa-induced dyskinesias in MPTP monkeys. Ann Neurol 2006; 59:282-288.

202. Santos-García D, Fonticoba TD, Cores Bartolomé C et al. Risk of cognitive impairment in patients with Parkinson's disease with visual hallucinations and subjective cognitive complaints. J Clin Neurol 2023 Jan 2. Online ahead of print.

203. Scalzo P, Kümmer A, Bretas TL et al. Serum levels of brain-derived neurotrophic factor correlate with motor impairment in Parkinson's disease. J Neurol 2010; 257:540-545.

204. Scammell TE, Arrigoni E, Lipton JO. Neural circuitry of wakefulness and sleep. Neuron 2017; 93:747-765.

205. Scandalis TA, Bosak A, Berliner JC et al. Resistance training and gait function in patients with Parkinson's disease. Am J Phys Med Rehabil 2001; 80:38-43.

206. Schneider RB, Lu X, Biglan K et al. Earlier dopaminergic treatment in Parkinson's disease is not associated with improved outcomes. Mov Disord Clin Pract 2019; 6:222-226.

207. Schenkman M, Moore CG, Kohrt WM et al. Effect of high-intensity treadmill exercise on motor symptoms in patients with *de novo* Parkinson's disease: a phase 2 randomized clinical trial. JAMA Neurol 2018; 75:219-226.

208. Schütz L, Sixel-Döring F, Hermann W. Management of sleep disturbances in Parkinson's disease. J Parkinsons Dis 2022; 12: 2029-2058.

209. Shen Y, Huang JY, Li J, Liu CF. Excessive daytime sleepiness in Parkinson's disease: Clinical implications and management. Chin Med J (Engl) 2018; 131:974-981.

210. Shih IF, Liew Z, Krause N, Ritz B. Lifetime occupational and leisure time physical activity and risk of Parkinson's disease. Parkinsonism Relat Disord. 2016; 28:112-117.

211. Siclari F, Valli K, Arnulf I. Dreams and nightmares in healthy adults and in patients with sleep and neurological disorders. Lancet Neurol 2020; 19:849-859.

212. Sleeman I, Aspray T, Lawson R et al. The role of vitamin D in disease progression in early Parkinson's disease. J Parkinsons Dis 2017; 7:669-675.

213. Small G, Vorgan G. Meet your ibrain. Scientific American Mind 2008; 19:42-49.

214. Smith AD, Castro SL, Zigmond MJ. Stress-induced Parkinson's disease: a working hypothesis. Physiol Behav 2002; 77:527-531.

215. Smith LK, Jadavji NM, Colwell KL et al. Stress accelerates neural degeneration and exaggerates motor symptoms in a rat model of Parkinson's disease.

216. Solms, M., and Panksepp J. The "id" knows more than the "ego" admits: neuropsychoanalytic and primal consciousness perspectives on the interface between affective and cognitive neuroscience. Brain Sci 2012; 2:147-175.

217. Soumyanath A, Denne T, Hiller A et al. Analysis of levodopa content in commercial *Mucuna pruriens* products using high-performance liquid chromatography with fluorescence detection. J Alt Complement Medicine 2018; 24:182-186.

218. Stevenson RL. *Virginibus puerisque* and other papers (1881). Translation: *Virginibus puerisque* y otros ensayos. Alianza, Madrid 1994.

219. Strandwitz P. Neurotransmitter modulation by the gut microbiota. Brain Res 2018; 1693(Pt B):128-133.

220. Suárez-García I, Gómez Cerezo JF, Ríos-Blanco JJ et al. Homocysteine: the cardiovascular risk factor of the next millennium? [Homocysteine. The cardiovascular risk factor of the next millennium?] An Med Interna (Madrid) 2001; 18:211-217.

221. Sun MF, Shen YQ. Dysbiosis of gut microbiota and microbial metabolites in Parkinson's disease. Ageing Res Rev 2018; 45:53-61.

222. Sun MF, Zhu YL, Zhou ZL et al. Neuroprotective effects of fecal microbiota transplantation on MPTP-induced Parkinson's disease mice: Gut microbiota, glial reaction and TLR4/TNF-α signaling pathway. Brain Behav Immun 2018; 70:48-60.

223. Suoh S, Donoyama N, Ohkoshi N. Anma massage (Japanese massage) therapy for patients with Parkinson's disease in geriatric health services facilities: Effectiveness on limited range of motion of the shoulder joint. J Bodyw Mov Ther 2016; 20:364-372.

224. Taghizadeh G, Azad A, Kashefi S, et al. The effect of sensory-motor training on hand and upper extremity sensory and motor function in patients with idiopathic Parkinson disease. J Hand Ther 2017; pii: S0894-1130(17)30004-2.

225. Tanaka K, Quadros AC Jr, Santos RF et al. Benefits of physical exercise on executive functions in older people with Parkinson's disease. Brain Cogn 2009; 69:435-441.

226. Thacker EL, Chen H, Patel AV et al. Recreational physical activity and risk of Parkinson's disease. Mov Disord 2008; 23:69-74.

227. Tillerson JL, Caudle WM, Reverón ME, Miller GW. Exercise induces behavioral recovery and attenuates neurochemical deficits in rodent models of Parkinson's disease. Neuroscience 2003; 119:899-911.

228. Tillerson JL, Cohen AD, Caudle WM et al. Forced nonuse in unilateral parkinsonian rats exacerbates injury. J Neurosci 2002; 22:6790-6799.

229. Tillmann AC, Andrade A, Swarowsky A, De Azevedo Guimarães AC et al. Brazilian Samba protocol for individuals with Parkinson's disease: A clinical non-randomized study. JMIR Res Protoc 2017; 6(7):e129. doi: 10.2196/resprot.6489.

230. Trappe HJ, Voit G. The cardiovascular effect of musical genres. A randomized controlled study on the effect of compositions by WA Mozart, J Strauss, and ABBA. Dtsch Arztebl Int 2016; 113:347-352.

231. Tvete IF, Klemp M. Parkinson's disease, treatment choice and survival over time. Clin Park Relat Disord 2022; 6:100136.

232. Valli K, Frauscher B, Peltomaa T et al. Dreaming furiously? A sleep laboratory study on the dream content of people with Parkinson's disease and with or without rapid eye movement sleep behavior disorder. Sleep Med 2015; 16:419-427.

233. Van der Giessen R, Olanow W, Lees A, Wagner H. Pharmaceutical compositions and uses comprising *Mucuna Pruriens* seed powder and extracts thereof in the treatment of neurological diseases. International Application published under the Patent Cooperation Treaty, 2004 13May. WO 2004/039385 A2, PCT/EP2003/010975. https://register.epo.org/ipfwretrieve?apn= JP. 2004547503. A&lng =en

234. Verschuur CVM, Suwijn SR, Boel JA et al, LEAP Study Group. Randomized Delayed-Start Trial of Levodopa in Parkinson's Disease. N Engl J Med 2019; 380:315-324.

235. Videnovic A, Klerman EB, Wang W et al. Timed light therapy for sleep and daytime sleepiness associated with Parkinson sisease: a randomized clinical trial. JAMA Neurol 2017; 74:411-418.

236. Walsh R. Lifestyle and mental health. Am Psychol 2011; 66:579-592.

237. Wang K, Li K, Zhang P et al. Mind-body exercises for non-motor symptoms of patients with Parkinson's disease: a systematic review and meta-analysis. Front Aging Neurosci 2021; 13:770920.

238. Wang W, Cui Y, Wen L et al. Dietary restriction against Parkinson's disease: what we know so far. Nutrients 2022; 14:4108.

239. Waterman D. Aging and memory for dreams. Perceptual and Motor Skills 1999; 73:355-365.

240. Wei W, Wang S, Xu C, et al. Gut microbiota, pathogenic proteins and neurodegenerative diseases. Front Microbiol 2022; 13:959856.

241. Willis GL, Turner EJ. Primary and secondary features of Parkinson's disease improve with strategic exposure to bright light: a case series study. Chronobiol Int 2007; 24:521-537.

242. Willis GL, Moore C, Armstrong SM. A historical justification for and retrospective analysis of the systematic application of light therapy in Parkinson's disease. Rev Neurosci 2012; 23:199-226.

243. Wirz-Justice A, Benedetti F, Terman M. Chronotherapeutics for affective disorders: A clinician's manual for light and wake therapy. S Karger AG, Basel 2013.

244. Wordsworth W, The world is too much with us. Poems, in two volumes (1807).

245. Wu PL, Lee M, Huang TT. Effectiveness of physical activity on patients with depression and Parkinson's disease: A systematic review. PLoS One 2017; 12: e0181515

246. Xie Y, Feng H, Peng S et al. Association of plasma homocysteine, vitamin B12 and folate levels with cognitive function in Parkinson's disease: A meta-analysis. Neurosci Lett 2017; 636:190-195.

247. Xu W, OuYang S, Chi Z et al. Effectiveness and safety of electroacupuncture in treating Parkinson disease. A protocol for systematic review and meta-analyses. Medicine (Baltimore). 2021 Mar 12; 100(10)

248. Yang CY, Kuo SH. Swimming with cerebellar ataxia. PM R. 2021; 13:425-426.

249. Yemula N, Dietrich C, Dostal V, Hornberger M. Parkinson's disease and the gut: symptoms, nutrition, and microbiota. J Parkinsons Dis 2021; 11:1491-1505.

250. Yogev-Seligmann G, Josman N, Bitterman N et al. The development of a home-based technology to improve gait in people with Parkinson's disease: a feasibility study. Biomed Eng Online 2023; 22:2.

251. Yoon SY, Suh JH, Yang SN et al. Association of physical activity, including amount and maintenance, with all-cause mortality in Parkinson disease. JAMA Neurol 2021; 78: 1446-1453.

252. Yuan S, Mason AM, Carter P et al. Homocysteine, B vitamins, and cardiovascular disease: a Mendelian randomization study. BMC Med 2021; 19:97.

253. Zanasi M, De Persis S, Caporali M, Siracusano A. Dreams and age. Perceptual and Motor Skills 2005; 100:925-938.

254. Zárate P, Díaz V. Music therapy applications in medicine. Rev Méd Chile 2001; 129:219-233.

255. Zesiewicz TA, Hauser RA. Sleep attacks and dopamine agonists for Parkinson's disease: what is currently known? CNS Drugs 2003; 17:593-600.

256. Zhang Y, Ren R, Sanford LD et al. Sleep in Parkinson's disease: A systematic review and meta-analysis of polysomnographic findings. Sleep Med Rev 2020; 51:101281.

257. Zhao Z, Ning J, Bao XQ, et al. Fecal microbiota transplantation protects rotenone-induced Parkinson's disease mice via suppressing inflammation mediated by the lipopolysaccharide-TLR4 signaling pathway through the microbiota-gut-brain axis. Microbiome 2021; 9:226.

258. Zheng L, Huiping QLe W et al. Vitamin D status and Parkinson's disease: a systematic review and meta-analysis. Neurol Sci 2014; 35:1723-1730.

259. Zhong Z, Chen W, Gao H, et al. Fecal Microbiota Transplantation Exerts a Protective Role in MPTP-Induced Parkinson's Disease via the TLR4/PI3K/AKT/NF-κB Pathway Stimulated by α-Synuclein. Neurochem Res 2021; 46:3050-3058.

260. Zhou Z, Zhou R, Zhang Z, Li K. The Association Between Vitamin D Status, Vitamin D Supplementation, Sunlight Exposure, and Parkinson's Disease: A Systematic Review and Meta-Analysis. Med Sci Monit 2019; 25:666-674.

261. Zhu M, Liu X, Ye Y, et al. Gut Microbiota: A Novel Therapeutic Target for Parkinson's Disease. Front Immunol 2022; 13:937555.

262. Zhuo C, Zhu X, Jiang R, Ji F, Su Z, Xue R, Zhou Y. Comparison for Efficacy and Tolerability among Ten Drugs for Treatment of Parkinson's Disease: A Network Meta-Analysis. Sci Rep *2017; 8:45865.* doi: 10.1038/srep45865.

263. Zoladz JA, Pilc A, Majerczak J et al. Endurance training increases plasma brain-derived neurotrophic factor concentration in young healthy men. *J Physiol Pharmacol* 2008; 59(suppl 7):119-132.

264. https://es.statista.com/estadisticas/590962/numero-de-muertes-por-parkinson-en-espana/

Table of contents

TABLE OF CONTENTS

Index 7
Introduction 9

1. Symptoms Dr. Parkinson never saw 13
   - AT 5 YEARS, NEW SYMPTOMS DUE TO DRUGS 13
   - HE "DANCES" BECAUSE OF TOO MANY PILLS 14
   - IN PRAISE FOR LEVODOPA 14
   - TOO MUCH CARBIDOPA ANTICIPATES DYSKINESIA 15
   - FEW DYSKINESIAS WITH LOW-DOSE LEVODOPA 16
   - AGONISTS ARE ANNOYING "ACOLYTES" 16
   - IS IT WORTH TWO YEARS ON AGONISTS? 17
   - CONSTIPATED, NIGHTMARES AND DAYTIME SLEEPINESS 18
   - TRAFFIC ACCIDENTS DUE TO AGONISTS 18
   - WATCH YOUR HEART AND BLOOD PRESSURE: MAOI ... 19
   - DOPAMINE DEMONS INVADE THE SHY PATIENT 20
   - IF HALLUCINATIONS, REMOVE ALL EXCEPT LEVODOPA 20
   - WHY DO PATIENTS NOW DIE EARLIER? 21
   - LABORATORIES PAY FOR CLINICAL TRIALS 22
   - IF A DRUG DID NOT IMPROVE YOU, QUIT IT 22

2. Brisk walking instead of Sinemet 25
    THE SOFA PREDISPOSES TO PARKINSON'S DISEASE 25
    EXERCISE SLOWS PARKINSON'S DISEASE 25
    BRISK WALKING (RAJOY'S MARCH) 26
    RAPID AND BRIEF VIGOROUS EXERCISE 26
    WALKING WITH MUSIC AND SMART GLASSES 27
    IF WALKING IS PAINFUL, IT'S TIME TO SWIM 27
    DYSKINESIAS ARE REDUCED BY SWIMMING 28
    THE "MOTOR MEMORY" OF GAIT 28
    ANY EXERCISE IMPROVES PATIENTS 29
    A GARDEN, A PARK, A FOREST 29
    CITIZENS HAVE DIVORCED FROM NATURE 30
    THE WISE HAVE A GARDEN 30
    TRUE TREATMENT IS A LIFESTYLE CHANGE[236] 31

3. I feel, therefore I exist 35
    SENSORY DIET 35
    FEELING IS LIFEBLOOD FOR THE BRAIN 36
    CHARCOT'S VIBRATORY CHAIR 36
    A TRACTOR RIDE BEFORE THE SINEMET 37
    STABILITY-ENHANCING VIBRATIONS 37
    SENSORY DISCHARGES IMPROVE MOTOR CONTROL ... 38
    KEEP YOUR FEET ON THE GROUND: "EARTHING". 38
    THUMB SUCKING AND TONGUE KISSING 39
    MASSAGE FOR PARKINSONIAN PATIENTS 39

AROMATHERAPY IN PARKINSON'S 39
THE BONBON IS A SENSORY LUXURY 40
MOZART REDUCES CORTISOL AND STRESS 41

4. Pleasure raises dopamine 43
PLEASURE IS A PRIMORDIAL FORCE 43
HEDONISM MEANS ENJOYMENT 44
THEY ENJOY LITTLE AND CONTROL A LOT 44
DR. FAUSTO GIVE UP STUDIES 45
PASSIONS AS THE YEARS GO BY 46
DIRTY OLD MEN DON'T GET PARKINSON'S DISEASE [79] . 46
THE PLEASURE MACHINE OF THE CRAZY PSYCHIATRIST' 47

5. Stress kills neurons 49
PSYCHOGENIC OR STRESS PARKINSONISM 49
MISMANAGING PROBLEMS 50
STRICT TEACHER, DEMANDING BOSS, NAGGING SPOUSE 51
ANTICIPATORY ANXIETY 51
I WRITE WHAT I SAW 52
CLASSICAL NEUROLOGISTS AND JUDGES BLAME STRESS 52
THE DANGER OF SUPPRESSING EMOTIONS 53
PARKINSON'S AS A CULTURAL DISEASE 54
SOCIETY AS A COLLECTIVE NEUROSIS 54

GET OUT OF THE HERD, ESCAPE THE SOCIAL NETWORK 55
COURT CONTEMPT AND HAMLET PRAISE[93] 56
THE CIMARRON BROKE HIS CHAINS................................ 56
THE POWER OF INSTINCT... 57
PSYCHOTHERAPY TO MANAGE STRESS 58

6. **Tell me your dreams and I'll predict your future 61**

LIFE IS A DREAM 61
DREAM CONTENT PREDICTS DISEASE COURSE 62
HYPNOS IS THE NIX SON AND THE ONYROS FATHER ... 62
OLD PEOPLE DREAM LESS 63
NIGHTMARES BEFORE PARKINSON'S 64
FURIOUS DREAMS AND ANIMAL AS PROTAGONISTS 64
SLEEP HEALS AND NOURISHES THE BRAIN 65
IF THE BRAIN SLEEPS BADLY, IT DEGENERATES 65
DON'T LET PILLS ROB YOUR DREAMS 66
SLEEP HYGIENE 67
NO ALARM CLOCK TO REMEMBER DREAMS 67
SUNBATHE TO GET A GOOD NIGHT'S SLEEP 68
MELATONIN ADJUSTS THE CIRCADIAN CLOCK 68
PHOTOTHERAPY TO RESTORE SLEEP RHYTHM............. 69

7. **Parkinson's disease is born in the gut 71**

SLOWER THE GUT, THE WORSE THE SYMPTOMS 71

PARKINSON'S DISEASE INVADES THE GUT	72
MICROBIOTA, CONSTIPATION AND PARKINSON'S DISEASE	72
MICROBIOTA, STRESS AND AGONISTS	73
BACTERIA "COOK" WHAT WE EAT	73
GUT IS A SOURCE OF DOPAMINE	73
DYSKINESIAS FROM DIGESTIVE ORIGIN	73
LEVODOPA'S EFFICACY DEPENDS ON WHAT YOU EAT	74
DIET IS PART OF TREATMENT	75
WITHDRAW DRUGS THAT CONSTIPATE YOU	75
PREBIOTICS AND PROBIOTICS	76
EAT LITTLE, WALK A LOT, AND LIVE LONGER	76
BRIEF INTERMITTENT FASTING	77
FAECAL TRANSPLANT AGAINST PARKINSON'S	78

8. Starting with natural levodopa (Mucuna) 81

THEY DESPISE THE MUCUNA THEY DON'T KNOW	81
SEED POWDER AND SEED EXTRACTS	82
MUCUNA IS BETTER THAN SINEMET OR MADOPAR	83
MUCUNA IS TOO EXPENSIVE WITHOUT CARBIDOPA	84
ZANDOPA IS THE CLINICAL TRIALS MUCUNA	85
GREEN TEA REINFORCES MUCUNA	85
ADDING CARBIDOPA TO MUCUNA	86
MUCUNA, SOYBEAN, ENTACAPONE, OPICAPONE, IMAO	86
FRAUDS WHEN BUYING MUCUNA	87

MUCUNA UPDATES 88

9. Mucuna for medicated patients 91
CHECK GENERAL MEDICATION 91
RECONSIDERING AGONISTS IN THE ELDERLY 92
LEVODOPA "AD LIBITUM", TO ECONOMISE IT 92
MUCUNA TO REPLACE SINEMET OR MADOPAR 93
MUCUNA ALONE WOULD BE VERY EXPENSIVE 93
MUCUNA USES THE CARBIDOPA OF SINEMET 94
CHECK THE INDIVIDUAL PROFILE FOR MUCUNA 94
HOW TO REDUCE SINEMET PLUS 25/100 (yellow) 95
HOW TO REDUCE MADOPAR 50/200 95
HOW TO REDUCE SINEMET 25/250 (blue) 96
MANAGEMENT OF THOSE TAKING STALEVO 96
DYSKINESIAS AND ADVANCED PATIENTS 97
MUCUNA CONTROLLED BY YOUR DOCTOR 97

10. Essential supplements 101
B6 FOR THOSE TAKING CARBIDOPA 101
B6, B9, B12 TO LOWER HOMOCYSTEINE 102
VITAMIN D DEFICIENCY IN THE ELDERLY AND
PARKINSONIANS 102
OMEGA 3 PREVENTS DYSKINESIAS 103
GREEN TEA 103
KEFIR AND PREBIOTICS 103
SLEEP SUPPLEMENTS 103

CAFFEINE AND GINSENG AGAINST DAYTIME DROWSINESS 104

ROYAL JELLY AND PROPOLIS 104

Epilogue 107
Bibliography 109
.... 110

Finis

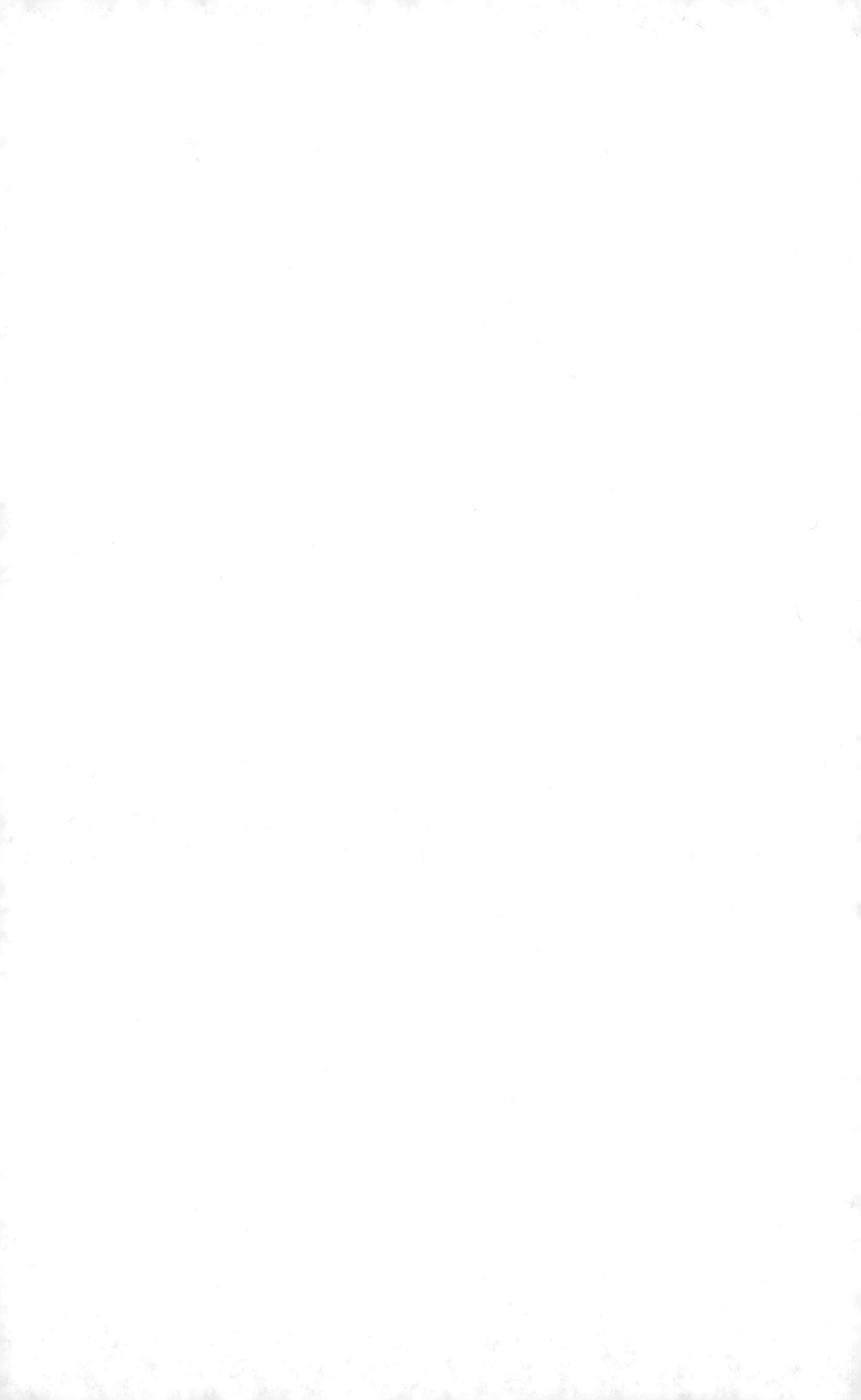

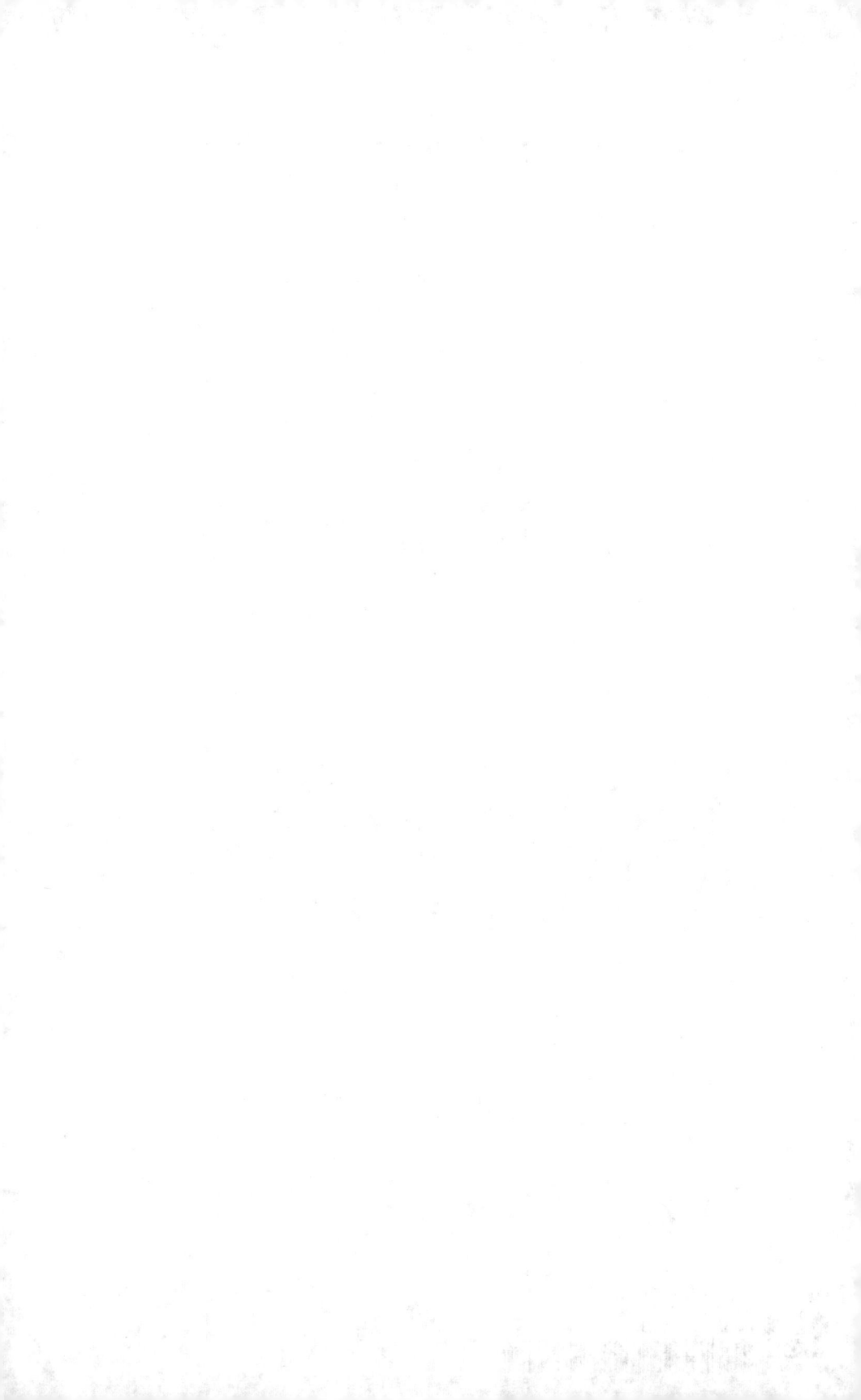

www.ingramcontent.com/pod-product-compliance
Lightning Source LLC
Chambersburg PA
CBHW050001230526
45465CB00003BB/1213